JAN KUPERMAN

DISABLED TO ABLE

From suffering to enlightenment

Disabled to Able: From suffering to enlightenment
© Jan Kuperman 2020

ISBN:
Paperback: 978-0-6451399-2-2
eBook: 978-0-6451399-1-4

A catalogue record for this book is available from the National Library of Australia

Original edit by Jacki Ferro of Raw Memoirs: www.rawmemoirs.com
Editors: Peta Culverhouse and Beverley Streater
Cover Design: Red Creative Design & Digital Pty Ltd
Original Design and Typeset: Ocean Reeve Publishing

Originally published by Jan Kuperman
www.jankuperman.com

Important Notes to the Reader

This book is intended as an informational guide. The remedies, approaches, and techniques described herein are meant to supplement, not be a substitute for, professional medical care or treatment. They should not be used to treat a serious ailment without prior consultation with a qualified health care professional.

Please note that some names have been changed to protect personal privacy.

Readers should also be advised that some material could cause distress. The author wants to present the views of many different healers and their healing modalities. She wishes to leave it up to the reader to decide what works best for them.

About the Author
Jan Kuperman

Jan's life has been filled with adventure and travel. Her family moved constantly from when she was seven and her childhood was spent moving from school to school. By the age of fourteen she'd attended twelve different schools. This upbringing brought with it the skills of adapting and a willingness to take a new path. A gypsy of sorts, her working life was also transient, with a range of diverse and varied jobs by the time she was 30 Jan found a great job working in a hospital where she unfortunately contracted two viruses simultaneously. This event, and her body's reaction, was what lead her on a harrowing path of pain and suffering Little did she realise then that this experience would leave her with a disability that would change her life. She faced a bleak future and was told she would become wheelchair bound for life. Through her determination to find the answers to regain her health, she began a journey of discovery outside the medical field. Jan would uncover new pathways and modalities where her own body, mind and spirit could begin to reverse the damage that was once thought to be irreparable.

Her book, *Disabled to Able - from suffering to enlightenment* is the story of her inspiring journey.

www.instagram.com/jankupermanGC
www.facebook.com/JanKupermanAuthor

Dedication

For those embarking on their own healing journey to wellness.
This has been my path; may it help guide you on your way.

Acknowledgements

I wish to acknowledge and thank all the healers who were there for me along this journey, and the friends I have made on this path of healing. A special thanks to the lovely ninety-year-old clairvoyant, Kawena, who first told me that I would be embarking on this writing journey, as impossible as I thought it was at the time.

To Gail, who read my first 10 000 words, and gave me some good advice. To Evie who, in the early days, when I was in a state of confusion about the whole process, listened and was caring and supportive during my phone calls. Her kind counsel kept me moving forward when I was ready to give in. Melissa, who suggested a new structure. My previous editor, Jacki, who has told me that she will now be learning Reiki. How good is that? Thank you—I was so emotional when you told me.

Big thanks to my husband, who sat down and read it in one afternoon and gave some good suggestions to my story.

Lastly, to all my family, a big thank you for all the good times.

Contents

Author's Note

My health problems have never defined me—I am a Pollyanna! I have always seen life as a glass half full. I can find a positive in a negative, and this attitude has helped me throughout my life.

Recently, I read this quote on a Facebook group page called *Love Wide Open*:

> I don't think anyone understands how tiring it is to act okay and always be 'strong' when, in reality, you're close to the edge. (anonymous)[1]

Personally, I live out the alternative to this way of thinking. I understand how tiring it can be to put on a brave face, but if you do keep putting on that brave face your body goes with you. Feeling up when you feel full of pain helps you through those days.

Over a year ago, I read a headline in the newspaper, "Industry mourns the loss of … " The woman who had died a world-renowned and talented artist, well-known to royalty, heads of state, and celebrities worldwide. After her cancer operation, she had been left with unbearable pain caused by nerve damage. A vibrant, funny, and creative woman, she had fallen to her death from a high-rise apartment and was now lost forever.

She was just sixty-two years of age and her suicide rocked me to my very core, as this wonderfully creative woman was someone my husband and I had met on occasion, joked with, and liked very much. Her loss of life resonated with me as I too have endured intense pain that goes for months on end. At times, I've felt close to the edge, and experienced a mindset where you can't even think straight from the pain. At the time, I wondered if she had explored alternative therapies.

This woman's death was one reason I have written this book. I want to share with sufferers of chronic pain that there are ways we can heal our bodies and our minds. The key lies in finding the therapy that resonates with you—be it acupuncture, hypnotherapy, EFT (Tapping) kinesiology, hydrotherapy, energy healing, homeopathy, essential oils, or one of the many others on offer. I have tried all these methods, and continue to use those I love still, as they all have a place in my ongoing healing. I hope that by sharing my story, I can help others reclaim their lives.

As Natalie Goldberg wrote in her book, *Old Friend from Far Away*:

> We write a memoir not to remember, not to cling, but to honour and let go.[2]

So here I am honouring and letting go.

Trying Times

It's April 2020 and we are in the midst of a worldwide pandemic. We are being told that the only way forward is to self-isolate. There is an old African saying that says, "It takes a village to raise a child." More than ever, we need to feel part of a community. From what I've seen on social media, I believe that this building of community is happening at a rapid rate. I have recently joined the Australian branch of Lynne McTaggart's Power of Eight group[3], sending good intentions out to the world.

Peaceful and loving thoughts bring about peaceful and loving results. At the moment, our world seems to be more fear-based. Who can blame us? We are being bombarded with negativity through the media at the most prime times of day, on both social media and through our home TV. At times, I have found this negativity overwhelming, and have needed to turn off the news bulletins.

Even our homegrown internationally known healer, shared with us this morning via social media that he had a small scare, thinking that he might have succumbed to the virus. After giving his body some rest, and releasing the fear, he is now at peace with the ongoing situation we all find ourselves in.

People have changed. They are now seeking ideas of how to help. I believe this shows that the fear is abating. We are living in a world that is all about increasing rates of isolation. One positive to come from this is that people are reaching out more and more, in many different ways, helping to raise each other's spirits which, in turn, improves our wellbeing.

From Able to Disabled
and Back Again

Way back in May of 1985, on a trip to visit an old family friend in Tasmania, I met two fascinating women. One was an old European lady, picking flowers in her garden, up in the hills behind Hobart. She was making and using Bach flower remedies. I learned that Bach remedies were made from the petals of flowers, distilled in water, and mixed with a small amount of brandy. These thirty-eight remedies were developed by homeopath Dr Edward Bach in the 1930s to gently heal a range of ailments and emotional issues. The other woman I met was helping a farmer's horse with back issues, using a form of hands-on energy healing from Japan. I was fascinated. At the time, I thought her work was a kind of chiropractic or massage treatment.

What further amazed me was that, through this energy therapy, this second woman was also helping the farmer to heal. Deformed and frozen by arthritis, the man was suffering constant pain. After watching, I asked for a session with her too. I was interested in feeling this in my own body what the farmer might have felt when receiving this magical energy. Little did I know that just a year later, I would personally experience the same chronic pain and restriction of movement, and endure deformities in my hands, fingers, and feet. Like this farmer, I would also find relief through energy healing.

During my years of disability, I often wondered what the purpose was of living a life so restricted and painful, especially as my life before had been so full of movement. Faith healing, the laying on of hands or spiritual healing, as it is called, was the dominant alternative healing tool practised in Australia during the 1980s. It was early in that decade too that Reiki was first introduced to Australia by American Reiki master, Beth Gray. In the mid-1980s, American author, Louise Hay, printed the first Australian edition of her short book, *You Can Heal Your Life* (1984). These healing therapies, modalities, and philosophies coincided with my own diagnosis of chronic arthritis.

Following a bike accident in 1986, American scientist, Joe Dispenza, was told he would never walk again. In his 2017 book, *Becoming Supernatural. How Common People are doing the Uncommon*, Joe explains how ordinary people can do the extraordinary, make enormous changes to their health, and reverse disease in their bodies. For me, this was a whole new way of thinking about the health and wellness of my mind and body.

We all have something to share and to offer, and everyone is here for a reason. This is my story of how, after living on an invalid pension for over three years, I overcame my disability, and returned to a fully functional and pain-free life. A psychiatrist and staff at my pain clinic had told me that I would be wheelchair-bound for the rest of my days. Like Joe Dispenza and many others, I didn't believe what I was told, and I looked for alternatives.

My dabble with being disabled (and I say dabble because it was only three years of restriction out of my life) led me on a path of trying many different and exciting healing methods. I read self-help books, attended seminars and workshops, for which I am so grateful. These learnings, and the people I have met along the way, have enriched my journey which I am still taking, and I would like to pass on what I have learnt.

Chapter 1

Chicken Feet for Hands

The first wealth is health.
—*Ralph Waldo Emerson*[4]

O ne morning, I couldn't move. My whole body felt trapped, as if locked inside a suit of armour. Lifting my hands to the light, they were contorted and looked like chicken feet.

I lay there for hours and grew increasingly frustrated. I lived alone, so no one was there to see me struggle. I thought then that having someone there would have been a great help.

So here I was, unable to move, but I needed to get out of this bed.

When, I had manoeuvred my legs over the side of the bed and stood up, half the day had passed. By then, who knew whether I had needed to be anywhere? I couldn't have cared less how important or otherwise any plans may have been. In previous weeks, this type of thing had happened occasionally, but it had never affected me for so long or so completely. The challenge and frustration gave the term "taking things slow" a whole new meaning for me. I felt like I was sinking into quicksand.

Large nodules protruded from every joint on every finger of both my hands, and they were swollen, red, and so painful. My once-nice hands with slim fingers now looked like twisted and ugly claws that were unrecognisable to me. It made me a little sad when I looked at them.

Once standing, the next goal was to find shoes to wear. My feet had swollen from my regular size seven and a half up to a size eight or at one time up to a nine which at first was quite alarming. I'd never know from one day to the next what size my feet would be. My shoes had to be ones that were easy to slip on and off.

I felt completely useless, as at times, I was unable to lift a phone or open my front door. Living in a ground floor flat, I had a sliding door that I often left unlocked as there was a short brick fence that I could clamber over, if things got a bit tricky and I needed an easy way in or out.

Walking had become a pain in more ways than one, but I used my cane for balance, most of the time to get from A to B. What I was also learning was patience. My body would completely seize up, and my muscles would say, 'No more walking for you today Miss.' I would find myself stationary for a while, stuck halfway up my street on the way to the shops for bread or milk. I would lean against the nearest fence and have my "stopping to smell the roses moment", as I would call it. Then, when I could, I would slowly saunter off again.

One time, a dear friend of mine, Heather, burst into tears seeing me trying to walk across a park with my cane. Even though it was very slow, I thought, *At least I'm walking*. That was the thought in my head, being forever the Pollyanna.

On mornings like this when I struggled to get out of bed, I thought, *So, this is how I live my life now ... waiting for the demise of my body.*

I was taking high doses of anti-inflammatories and I relied on gadgets to help me get throughout the day. One helped me put on my socks and shoes. Another helped me to open bottles and jars, and another was my cane that kept me balanced and supported when I walked or climbed stairs. All these items had become a part of my life, and I found them wonderfully helpful and, at times, so necessary. Back then, a mobile phone would have been a great addition too. The phone that I had was too heavy at times to lift and forget about dialling the numbers.

Friends would come to visit, and at times my hands were so twisted that I couldn't turn the front doorknob to let them in. They would then do I as did, and step over the small brick wall of my patio, coming in through the sliding door at the back, which I left unlatched.

My friends were my lifeline as my immediate family were living thousands of miles away.

Yet, throughout all this restriction and pain, I found the positives. After my years of living like a nomad without a home base, my illness was forcing me to stay still. And the pluses that came with that were enormous. After years of unpredictability and restlessness, in a weird way, I felt that I had found stability, constancy, and a sense of calm.

Before my condition, I had kept diaries for every single year of my life. During those three years, however, when the pain in my hands was far too strong to possibly bother, I did not keep up with my diaries. Unfortunately, I have little documentation of these three years. I could hardly hold a pen at times, let alone write lengthy diary entries. What I have kept is a medical notice of referral to a specialist from a doctor at the Alfred Hospital stating that I was a 31-year-old invalid pensioner. The letter was dated December 2, 1987.

Chapter 2

A Lifetime of Symptoms

Go confidently in the direction of your dreams,
live the life you imagined.
—Henry David Thoreau[5]

As a four-year-old living in the UK, I was staying with my mother's parents for a short time, as my parents had separated.

The backdoor stairs to the garden were very steep for me as I was quite short. I still am. One day, I took a tumble and landed face-first on a broken tile that was sticking up from the path below. The tile split open my forehead. Nana May rushed out to me, bundled me up and took me to her neighbour who had studied first aid. He took one look at my head and rushed my grandmother and myself to hospital. As the doctor stitched up my head, I didn't cry. I was being brave and strong. I remember Mum sitting beside my bed, holding my hand, and telling me how brave I was. Mum was working fulltime. I remember being so proud of my scar. I wore it as a badge of honour for the good and brave girl I was. This marked the beginning of my trying to prove how strong and resilient I was for Mum.

Thinking back now, I wonder if this childhood fall was the start of my path along the road to illness, and how I learned to deal with it. They say that your first seven years of life are so important. For me, these formative years were disrupted.

After my parents' brief separation, they reconciled, but two years later, at the age of seven, I was taken to a different country, away from my school, my family, and my friends—far away from all the people and places I had loved all of my life—those who had formed my world.

Our move resulted from my baby brother becoming very ill. At six months of age, after enduring a freezing cold winter, Dave had developed a dangerous chest infection. An Australian doctor suggested to Mum that he needed a warmer climate. 'Otherwise,' the doctor said, 'you might lose him to another winter.'

Mum had experienced the Battle of Britain where everyone had to queue for food rations. Often, she had told us stories of her childhood. 'One of my favourite memories was when I was a girl during the Battle of Britain,' Mum said. 'I remember queuing for these delicious, Australian navel oranges. The taste was amazing! Everything was rationed, and these were such a treat. I never stopped imagining what Australia must be like, with trees filled with these beautiful fruits.'

The sweet taste of those oranges stayed with Mother throughout her childhood and into adulthood so, when the doctor suggested a warmer climate, she immediately thought of Australia. *Australia! This would be a fantastic adventure!*

We left England on a beautiful ship called the Oriana. A trip by sea to Australia at that time cost £120, but because of the Assisted Passage Migration Scheme looking for workers and to increase the population, Mum and Dad only paid £10 each, and we kids came for free. Few could afford the full cost of the fare. When Mum and Dad landed, they only had £20 to live on. Migrants had to promise to stay for two years or pay the £110 difference. Quite a few of Australia's music legends came over in this way. We all know about the Bee Gees, but there were others, including Red Symons from the Skyhooks.

We had left home with very little, and Mum and Dad knew that I was missing family, so on the voyage over they wanted to buy me a doll. Something just for me to have of my own, as a birthday gift. While we were in port in Italy, they found a beautiful Italian doll with dark hair and vibrant clothes. She was gorgeous. But I didn't want her. I wanted a bride doll. My parents were a bit disappointed, but we carried on our journey. We docked at the port of Yemen where Dad wanted to buy souvenirs. Dad and I boarded a little boat and we were winched down the side of the ship into the sea before landing onshore. Off we went through the noisy streets. I found my doll in the markets of Aden, of all places! A red-headed, beautiful doll in a white bridal dress and veil.

Mum still has a photo of me sitting at the bottom of some stairs on the ship clutching onto my bride doll. When I look back, I can see that this doll was the very image of my aunty who we had left behind in the UK. I was obviously missing family, even if I didn't understand my feelings back then. As I grew older, I realised that what I wanted was to connect with home. The boat trip was a long journey of more than three weeks, and I was homesick. I needed something familiar.

When we finally docked in the port of Melbourne, we were handed coloured buttons. These buttons indicated where our bus would take us to our new home. We were accommodated in the Broadmeadows Housing Barracks or hostel—as they called it—a former army barracks. We lived in a tin hut behind gates that were closed at night, but hey, beggars can't be choosers.

I am not saying that moving to Australia was the wrong thing to do—quite the opposite, especially for my brother. However, boarding that ship and leaving everyone and everything behind that I knew, did have an impact on me. For one thing, arriving in our new homeland saw the start of my eczema. Rashes covered my hands and parts of my body. The itchiness was unbearable, and Mum would often put socks on my hands to stop me from clawing at my skin. I told myself to be strong and to not complain.

On our arrival in June 1963, while our little family lived in that hostel, both my parents worked. I started at a primary school nearby and, after school, I babysat my younger baby brother and sister, Julie. Always working, because they had to, Mum and Dad bought me a TV to watch to help me cope, but my skin rashes grew out of control. Dad was highly intelligent. He had studied at Oxford University and, after we migrated, he also attended night school. He was very much of the old school where children were seen and not heard. My parents then paid a Dutch lady who lived in the hostel to look after my six-month-old brother, eighteen-month-old sister, and me, when I came home from school. I no longer had that responsibility, and this quite possibly saw an end to my skin breakouts. My parents worked constantly to put food on the table. We had arrived with nothing, and our furniture was very basic.

I desperately wanted to make friends to fill the void of loneliness. One day, I had a great idea to swap our souvenirs from the trip with the kids in the hostel. *I will make lots of friends!* I thought.

When my parents arrived home and discovered what I had done, they weren't happy. *Seriously not happy, Jan.* That evening, Dad marched me around to every tin hut. I had to apologise to each family and return everything I had swapped. I felt humiliated and small. I wanted to hide away. It's one of the things that I wished I didn't remember as I became an adult, but it was something that was not forgiven or laughed away, and so it stayed with me in my memory and in my body. To this day, Mum has not forgiven me for swapping her Spanish knitting patterns that were never returned as we had so little.

During our initial year, Mum and Dad continuously moved for work, so I had to attend two different schools in a short time. We moved from the hostel to live in Melbourne city after my parents and another English family, from the barracks—the two Mums had met over the concrete troughs where they did the family washing—decided to pool their wages and rent a house together. We were two families of four adults and five kids living in a four-bedroom house. Three kids bunked in one room and two in the other bedroom, while the parents took the remaining two rooms. It wasn't ideal, but I now had a new extended family with a new aunty and uncle. It was only for a short time, but at least we were out of the hostel where some families lived for years. Mum and Dad didn't want that for us kids and feared we might get stuck there. We stayed in contact with this family all our lives, and Mum and her best friend still talk on the phone.

Whinging Poms

I recently read an article called *Post World War II British Migration to Australia* by Celia Pullen. In it, Celia writes:

> For those who were lucky enough to have existing family in Australia or for those who were nominated by an Australian company or citizen, accommodation was usually sorted before they arrived. However, for the majority emigrating with no connections and often little funding, they found themselves in migrant hostels in arriving in Australia. Hostel conditions left much to be desired, from most accounts, providing only basic living arrangements, usually set up in former Nissan huts used during the war
>
> The British migrants that complained about hostel conditions soon obtained the nickname, 'Whingeing

Poms,' which became a source of mockery for many Australians who encountered the new arrivals. [6]

I have always wondered where that term had come from because my family were the exact opposite. They had been given an opportunity and they were running with it. The way to do that was to get the hell out of Dodge. Sorry, I meant to say ... to get the hell out of the hostel.

*

A couple of months later, I was moved to and attended four different schools while still aged seven. These massive changes were a lot to process for a little kid but, in those times, no one asked if you were coping when you were that age.

After I turned eight, we moved to Sunbury, forty kilometres inland from Melbourne. Our house was in the country and unlike anything else we had seen so far. It was more like a shack and was a bit of a shock for a family who was used to living in the well-established and bustling major city of London. With weatherboard walls, our new home was one step up from the tin hut we had endured at the hostel. Our lives became dusty, dry, and hot, and we had very little furniture. We sat on crates, but Mum was enterprising, setting up her ironing board as a dinner server. This was all good fun to us kids.

Our only toilet was a long-drop outhouse, a substantial walk away from the house through the tall grass. It was a simple, small shed with a hole in the ground, and the blowflies were horrendous, buzzing around constantly. The swarms were thick enough to throw a sandwich in for them to eat whole. I look at the show *I'm a Celebrity, Get Me Out of Here* and laugh. Been there, done that! We didn't end up staying long. Years later, Sunbury would become well known for its music festivals, probably with better toilets than ours.

As far as I remember, we moved from Sunbury back to the city where we lived in a two-storey townhouse. Shortly after, my other nan, Dad's mum, Nana Mobbs, arrived from London to live with us. Until Nana Mobbs arrived, aside from that brief stint under the care of the Dutch woman, I had been the chief babysitter for my younger brother and sister. I was known as a latchkey kid, left alone to look after myself.

A year later, we moved again, to another bushland area. This time, however, we were nestled in lush, green country, near Eltham in outer Melbourne. I had great fun there, and even learned how to ride a horse, and I made some great friends. But we didn't stay for long as we were renting, and the owner was wanting to move back.

My life became a set of revolving doors. We moved to Sandringham, or "Sandy" as it was called, walking distance to the beach. This time, our house was draughty, and falling down in places. There were holes in the roof, and I was electrocuted while there. Dad was trying to fix the big, round Bakelite light switch in the front room. He hadn't finished fixing it, and huge copper wires stuck out from the wall. I reached around the wall to flick on the switch. Hitting only wires, I was thrown across the room and ended up seeing stars. What a shock! My hand was burned, but I didn't go to a doctor or hospital. We bandaged it up and life went on.

This, of all places, was the one house where we stayed for a couple of years. It wasn't ideal, but at least it was stable. Sandy was and still is a charming area, and I loved it there. After my hand healed, I was fit, healthy, and happy. One of our most famous prime ministers, Bob Hawke, lived in the area too. This was where I learnt to swim at the beach. Mum was working two jobs during the week, and Sundays at the zoo, taking the entrance fees. I loved going there and spending time with her. I finished state school and had two great years at Hampton high school where I made some great friends and I was hoping to become a teacher, I loved it so much. You can guess what happened next ... Yep, another move. This time we settled into a beach house at Rye on the Mornington Peninsula. This was the first house my parents purchased; those six years of hard work had paid off. It was a lovely place and our house sat among the sand dunes, surrounded by bushland. At this time, life was fun and carefree. We would listen to the sound of waves crashing as we fell asleep. This was more in line with what my parents had thought Australia would be like and, although it was a three-mile walk to catch the bus to high school, I enjoyed our relaxing lifestyle.

Every year, a carnival came to the shorefront and the three of us had fun learning to shoot the metal ducks on the firing range. At the end of the school holidays, as the carnival was packing up to leave, my brother and sister would race around to collect the fallen coins.

By this time, I was a teenager working in a milk bar after school and on weekends to earn pocket money. I felt more comfortable working this job than I did learning in the classroom where I was always the new girl, trying to make friends. When I turned fourteen, I worked for the Bar 20 Horse Ranch, helping to bring in the horses for people to ride on weekends.

Later, my parents bought me a horse of my own. I called him Brigadoon. The money I earned working weekends went into buying his saddle and keeping him in feed. Brigadoon was beautiful, but he was huge, standing fifteen hands tall. An ex-pacer, Brigadoon would buck me off his back as if I was an annoying fly. A quick twitch and I was left sitting on my backside on the gravel by the side of the road. I took so many falls from the ages of nine to sixteen, it's a wonder that nothing ever got broken. Lucky for me, I bounce. One time, Brigadoon was spooked and galloped down the road with me barely hanging on.

Cars driving past were giving me a wide berth. Eventually, he ran out of steam enough for me to slip off. I walked him back home—my legs like jelly. After that, I grew scared of riding him and the original owner took him back.

Besides my horse, we kept many different animals—dogs, cats, birds, foxes, everything made up our menagerie of rescue animals and their friends. One day, we rescued a racing greyhound who was about to be put down by the local trainer up the road. Tuddie would let off the most horrendous farts. He also had a thing for backsides and would nip at holiday-makers as they jogged along the roadside.

Sadly, while we lived there, Nana Mobbs passed away in her late seventies from bowel cancer. So, I became the babysitter once more, and the idea of earning a full-time wage became increasingly more appealing to me than schoolwork and so, I left school for good.

At fifteen, I was working for the local newsagent. As history repeats, I didn't last there long. Next, I got a job working in a fashion shop called *The Jean Keeper* and I was now sixteen nearly seventeen years old. Later, I took over as manager. I had lied about my age, telling the owner that I was eighteen. I had a good group of friends, a career I now loved, and a nice boyfriend. Here we were living the quintessential Aussie lifestyle—our back garden was a surf beach, our nearest neighbour lived a mile down the road, the air was clean, and the skies were blue. By this stage too, more of our family from England, including my Aunty Irene, Uncle Tony, and cousins, had emigrated and lived close by. Everything was going great, and I was happily settled.

But then my grandad in England died, and Nana May wanted us to return to live with her. Dare I say it? There was a pattern emerging. I wanted to stay, but we were such a close-knit family unit. Dad was offered a one-year contract with an oil company, so we thought it would be exciting. A decade after we had sailed halfway around the world to live in Australia, we left, and found ourselves living back in London.

For me, returning turned out to be another culture shock. London was so busy—there were people everywhere. Here we were now, these quiet country kids from Australia, and the clamour of London was overwhelming. The trains were noisy, and everything looked grey. It was the era when young people dressed as goths, and young shop assistants at Biba scared me a bit, I felt like a country bumpkin. The mid-70s were the time of the IRA bombings, and all the tourist spots were being targeted. Luckily for us, our angels were watching, and we missed all these bombings by visiting these hotspots at different times. We dodged the 1974 bombing of Madame Tussauds and the Tower of London by only a few hours. Both Mum and Dad grew up as children of the Battle of Britain, so the IRA bombing terror was not easy for them to endure. But "life goes on" was Mum's motto, so we didn't stop our sightseeing.

On our return to England, my younger siblings, Julie and Dave, were bullied quite a lot by the English children, as they were the Aussie kids with funny accents.

When we first settled back into London life, Dad worked on two, one-year contracts for an oil company in the North Sea.

We had only been there a short time when, aged seventeen, I started working for a company called Honeywell, doing key tape data entry. My new role was a huge change from that of a clothing manager with a staff of one. I was now employed by a massive company with its staff of thousands.

One afternoon, as I headed home after work, my bus pulled into the stop across the highway. The driver in the nearest lane to me waved me across, so I started to walk towards my ride. Unseen by me, a second car was coming up fast alongside the first. I didn't see him, and he didn't see me, until I hit the front of his bonnet. I can remember feeling very embarrassed as my co-workers from Honeywell would have seen me sprawled across the road.

I was taken to St Bartholomew's Hospital, but sent home as they were short of beds, and my accident wasn't life-threatening. The men in my family had to carry me up and down the stairs because, for a time, I couldn't walk. That incident left me with fatty tissue on my thigh that was the size of an Aussie Rules football. This was my first experience of being incapacitated in any way.

After this road accident, I started to see clairvoyants, as I didn't want to be blindsided again, literally.

In 1975, there was another move. We moved from North London to South London, to a place called Weybridge. This time, I didn't mind the change. Weybridge was gorgeous, countrified, and very picturesque. Our rented house in a huge private estate sat on the river, and even came with a grand piano in the lounge room. Cliff Richard lived close by, and The Beatles once lived there too. We had ducks and swans that would come to the backdoor squawking to be fed. There was also a squirrel that my brother named, Peanuts, that came up to the house … yes, to be fed his peanuts. Dad was still working for the oil company and travelling overseas quite a bit, so Mum and I thought it might be fun to apply for work together. We were glad we did.

My next role would be my fourth job in the UK and the eighth of my working career so far. I was just eighteen years old. I went for what was the highest paying job at the time. I didn't care what it was. My job at a factory up the road paid thirty pounds a week, and it was fun. This was no ordinary factory. There were a wonderful group of women working there, from all different backgrounds. Catholics worked happily alongside Protestants. This was the time when the Irish were bombing the UK, yet all these women got on like a house on fire and were very understanding of each other's religion. I soon fell for an Irishman who also worked there.

Dad had come to the end of his second-year contract. Although I was about to be promoted to the pathology section of the factory, it was time to move, again. Leaving that beautiful town and our large house on the estate, not to mention my Irish guy, was heartbreaking. But my life's pattern was repeating itself. I could have stayed but, in the end, I chose the love of a country and my family over a dear, sweet guy.

Back to Australia we came.

In 1976, we arrived back on the Mornington Peninsula in Victoria. This time, my parents bought a house close to where we had lived before leaving for London—back to the sun, sand and sea. We filled our home with dogs, cats, chooks, and birds, our usual menagerie. Our friends from before we had left, again became regular visitors, and life flowed on.

Unfortunately, not long after we settled in, my parents had to move to the city for work. They left my siblings and me behind in the beach house. I was now twenty years old and looking after a disgruntled fifteen-year-old sister who was having to put up with her older sister being in charge, and a fourteen-year-old, wayward little brother who enjoyed joy-riding with some older boys in the neighbourhood. Who could blame them? I think we were all a little lost.

Things became better for all when Mum and Dad took my teenage siblings to the city to live with them, leaving me to run my own show. I worked hard and found myself a new job. Later that year, the beach house was sold, and I too moved to the city. Three jobs later, Dad was posted interstate to Sydney.

What could we all do but pack up as a family and move to Sydney? So, that was that. We were on the move yet again.

Chapter 3

Starting and Stopping

Believe you can and you're halfway there.
—*Theodore Roosevelt*[7]

Once in Sydney, in my early twenties, I worked three different jobs at the same time. I was a casual for Soccer Pools that later became Lotto, and, at one stage, I drove an old London taxicab. It was great fun. My second job was doing bar work in a hotel and, on the weekends, I booked caravans for a motorhome hire company.

One of my favourite roles came next, working as a reservations clerk for the Sebel Townhouse Hotel. I had a new guy in my life, and his lovely mum gave me a full-time position working with her. It was an exciting time to be working there as all the most famous names stayed at the Sebel when performing in Sydney. I was lucky enough to meet a few—The Doobie Brothers, Billy Joel, John McEnroe, and The Village People—that created quite a stir when they stayed there in 1980. It was such an excellent place to work that I never thought I would have to leave.

However, inconsistency had been my life for so long that I had grown comfortable with it, and I had no idea how to live any differently. Friends, boyfriends, work associates, and workplaces were never long-time considerations. I had never known anything to remain permanent, apart from my immediate family. Living in Sydney with a fantastic job, however, I began to learn that it was safe for me to stay in one place. Before then, safety to me involved movement, change, lack of direction, and going with the flow.

Life in Sydney was fun. After work, I took an evening dance class. From there I went ice skating, then finished off the night with a run. After a few weeks though, my leg was starting to ache, but I thought it was from overuse. The enormous lump of dead, fatty tissue, leftover from the car accident in the UK, still bulged from my right leg. While it hadn't bothered me previously, apart from cutting a less than flattering silhouette in tight skirts, now it had really started to ache, so I decided that I could ignore it no more. The pain had also started to restrict me from doing many things, so I thought I should see a doctor.

The doctor took one look at my thigh and told me he was worried I had cancer. He wanted it tested immediately, and he took a biopsy. Lucky for me, the test came back benign, but the lump was removed regardless. The surgery went well, but it left a deep indentation in my thigh and two decent-sized scars. Again, tight skirts would never look quite right on me, but at least I could now do yoga, and maybe go horse-riding again—all good and positive things. I was twenty-four and, while the lump had given me a scare when I'd thought I could have cancer and lose my leg, my overriding thought was that life can be short, so I should enjoy every minute.

When I returned home from hospital, my work colleague was heading off to Europe and, after my health scare, I decided to go with her. It was March,1982. Our grand adventure took us to Greece, France, Amsterdam, and finally Germany where I left my friend, and went on to the UK. Travelling on my own was challenging, but I met terrific people along the way, and I loved my time in Europe. The only niggling thing going on with me was repeated bouts of stomach upset. I thought my discomfort might have come from the food market stalls on the different Islands we had visited in Greece.

Back in the UK, I found my way to a backpacker-style hotel called The Colonial Club. It was there that I met a girl named Anne, from Melbourne, who was also keen to travel around the UK. I was short on money, arriving with only £65 pounds in my pocket, but luckily a friend who I had worked with in Sydney let me stay bunking in with her and her flatmates.

It was my twenty-fifth birthday, yet I had heard nothing from my family. To say I was disappointed is an understatement. Five days later, Anne and I took off on our three-week trip around England, Wales, and Scotland. We hired a car, planning to stop wherever we liked. We drove along coastal roads, dropping in on villages with cobbled roads and tree-covered lanes, and hedges so high you felt like you were driving through a winding maze.

Glastonbury and the Abbey in Somerset were particular highlights. Walking through the grounds of the Abbey, I fell to my knees and said to Anne, 'Leave me here.' I felt such a connection, a pull to that place, and I didn't want to leave; it felt like I had come home.

Of course, I could not have stayed in Glastonbury, but that memory, that feeling, stayed with me, almost haunted me and I never forgot it. Returning to London, we booked a trip to Portugal together as a way of relaxing after our fun but exhausting journey around the UK. Once again, we discovered a stunning country. Sitting at a little café on the beach, I ate a plate of sardines the size of my feet that I had watched the local fishermen catch earlier that morning. Portugal was a succession of beautiful beaches, one after the other, and the food was fresh and tasty—I loved eating the fish—I was, still dealing with bouts of an upset tummy, but I put it down to the different water and the change in diet. While my digestive problems had been happening for three or four months, nothing stopped me from eating, that's for sure. I was such a lover of my food.

On returning to London, I had received a letter from home, and then I got a phone call from Mum. All was well.

Arriving back home to Sydney in August 1982, my family were waiting for me at the airport. It was a lovely homecoming. I moved in with my family and found a job straight away. Things were not good at home and I could feel the tension all around me. Mum and Dad were not talking, and Mum had decided to leave. This was the last time my family would be together as one unit.

Soon after my return, both Julie and Dave left Sydney, also looking for adventure. Dave applied for a job in Katherine in the Northern Territory. Later, Mum and I followed, and soon my family started work at a million-acre cattle and small crop station, living in a caravan that my brother had bought with his earnings. The only other accommodation options were dongas, which were there for the single male workers, and were basically a one-room transportable hut.

My family loved life in the outback. Vast, red dust surrounded us, and at night we would sit back and watch the storms come over. Storms are phenomenal in the outback because it's all so open, even the stars seem more spectacular. For a few weeks, while working out what to do next, I stayed with my family in the caravan. One day, I put my hand up to help in the kitchen, as the cook had to go to hospital. I thought I knew what I was doing as I had been cooking for years. I decided to make them all beef casserole. *Easy peasy*, I thought. But then I asked where the fridge was. I was pointed in the direction of a cold room. I had never been inside a cold room before. I got the shock of my life. Vast carcasses of blackened meat hung from huge hooks. Generally, for me, meat came from the butchers, looking all pretty, pink, portioned, and named. I had no idea where to cut the meat, so I just sliced off the nearest chunk. I think it turned out to be topside. It became a very expensive casserole. Luckily, that was my only stint there as relief cook. While my family loved living on the station, being hot, dusty, and miles from anywhere, it wasn't for me.

I was out of funds, so I ventured up to Darwin to earn enough money to fly back to Sydney. While staying in a backpackers' hostel there, I became great friends with an easy-going and very caring nurse, Bree, from Adelaide. We drove the three-and-a-half hours south to Katherine to meet my family, and then drove on so that I could show Bree Katherine Gorge. We ended up staying in the town of Katherine and sharing a unit.

Whilst Katherine is not a large town, it is large on character. Points of interest include the supermarket where, local legend has it, a giant crocodile was found munching through the meat counter after flood waters subsided in 1998. Katherine is also a crossroads town, linking many outback routes from Queensland, Western Australia, and the Northern Territory. The town is better known for the Nitmiluk National Park a beautiful natural oasis (formerly Katherine Gorge). This majestic site contains thirteen impressive deep gorges that wind their way through ancient limestone cliffs up to 70 metres tall and follow along the Katherine river.

Bree found a job at the hospital, and I went to work for the Katherine Gorge Tourist Agency. This was to be the most interesting of all my jobs so far. One day, while pumping petrol, I met Priscilla Presley as I fuelled up her limo. I was taken aback that Priscilla was being chauffeured around the Top End, just her and her driver. We had a brief chat. She was warm and friendly. The people you meet in outback Australia!

I filled gas bottles for the campers, sold souvenirs in the gift shop, which I also vacuumed and dusted, and took bookings for the evening shows and walks through Katherine Gorge. I also made reservations for the Greyhound Bus: a "Jill of all Trades".

Not long after starting to enjoy life in Katherine, my friend learned that she had contracted hepatitis. Bree had to fly home to Adelaide, and that meant I could not afford to stay where I was living. So, out to the gorge I went. The staff there were fantastic, like one big happy family. I went out with the tours up the gorge, and I was also a fast-food cook, flipping burgers over a hot plate for the busloads of tourists. I got so hot cooking that sweat ran down my nose and dropped onto the hotplate, sizzling and spitting. *Extra salt with those egg and bacon burgers anyone?* I also helped with the rubbish run—an Emu-bobber—as the garbage collector was known. I have a photo of me driving this old truck with a big grin on my face.

A cute little dingo often came into the grounds where I worked. Someone named him Socks. Socks often chased one of the resident emus around the trees. It was gorgeous to watch. They played peekaboo around the tree trunks. It was the funniest thing. Joeys (what young kangaroos are called), came into our vans and hopped onto the beds. The guy I was now living with, in a caravan, would feed the little joeys his cereal. This was a fantastic time in my life. I loved being that close to all the wildlife. While there, an old friend I had worked with at the Sandringham Hotel in Melbourne got in touch. Cherub, so named by my family because she looked like an angel, with blonde hair and blue eyes, suggested we meet in Bali for a holiday.

As you might have guessed by now, I am never one to say no to travelling.

In Bali, Cherub and I stayed in both Legian and Ubud. Back then, Ubud was nothing like the tourist mecca that it is now. I have been back there twice in recent years and can't get used to how bustling it has become. *Is this what we call progress?* Cherub and I went from the sublime to the ridiculous. Legian provided huge rooms and luxury, while Ubud was grotty, and the toilets involved standing over a cement hole to wee. It was Sunbury revisited, but without the giant blowflies. I ate from the side stalls and developed what I thought was a touch of Bali Belly.

It was towards the end of the trip I was taken to a German doctor. He told me to return home immediately. Luckily, I was flying out the next day. My guy came to Darwin and collected me from the airport. I have photos of me looking tanned, happy, and plump from good eating. But this didn't last long. Soon I ended up in our local hospital where I stayed for ten days.

I had ingested an amoeba called E. histolytica. I was bloated and suffering huge tummy upsets and unable to do much. Apparently, this parasite had been with me for a while, travelling the world with me since Greece. Doctors had a hard time finding this bug, but they were eventually able to remove the freeloader from my stomach, but not before I had lost a lot of weight. By the time I was discharged, I looked gaunt, and my bones stuck out everywhere. But I had stunning cheekbones and lovely shoulder blades—a little plus for my troubles, and my boyfriend loved my new look. *Win-win!*

It was the end of the tourist season in Katherine. The wet season would soon start, so my guy drove us to Townsville to look for work. My troubles were not over. That little bug had done some damage and, although I was living in one of the most gorgeous cities in Queensland, I continued to feel ill. I knew something was not right and kept returning to the doctor. The doctor I saw eventually blamed my sickness on having an overly active sex life! *Huh?*

Two months after arriving in Townsville, while getting out of our Land Cruiser, I collapsed onto the footpath and was rushed to hospital. They found that I had gangrene of the bowel. My stomach was opened, and they operated to remove the infection immediately. I awoke to find that the surgeons had stapled my tummy together. A long row of metal staples ran down the length of my stomach. *So not sexy, Doc!*

Shortly after I was discharged and the staples were taken out, I was shocked one day to see my stomach starting to open. The wound had not held together. But there was no way I was going back to that hospital. So, I grabbed some plasters, and taped myself up. *There you go ... all done.* I have to admit that the scar that I was left with was not so good. Soon after, my guy and I split, he returned to Katherine and I moved into a caravan at the local campsite. I met a lovely Kiwi girl and we became friends, and I got a good job working as a trainee manager at the Travelodge Hotel. My mum, brother, my sister, and her husband had also left Katherine and moved to Townsville. When they arrived, we decided to rent a house together and, for a while, things were going well. It was lovely to have my family together under one roof.

I enjoyed living in Townsville. They say that, living there, you can have an outdoor BBQ every month of the year, but one. And it was true. For the entire month of January, it rained heavily.

The pattern of my life was to carry on through.

A few months later, my sister and brother-in-law left to live with his family down closer to the Whitsundays, an absolutely stunning part of the world. My brother also moved out to live with his girlfriend who he had met through me, and eventually married. A manager from the station who was in love with my mum drove to Townsville, collected Mum, and took her back to live with him in Katherine where they ended up building a house together.

I was left wondering what the hell had happened. For some reason, I decided to head home. I was now twenty-nine years of age, alone, and feeling unsure of what to do next. Although I had moved around a lot and lived in many different cities, towns, and even countries, home to me was where I had spent my childhood, and where I had learnt to ride wild horses.

I packed up my car and drove south. But then my car had a slight hiccup in Sydney. I decided to travel the rest of the way to Melbourne by train. It was more enjoyable for both me and my car.

Initially, I rented a room for a short time from a lovely lady who introduced me to the joys of cross-country skiing. Little did I know that this lady would also be the one to point me in the direction of my healing.

Shortly after arriving, a good friend from Townsville joined me in Melbourne, and we moved into a flat together. I soon felt a need to find out why I was so confused with life—I was feeling lost and with no direction. I had spent years trying to keep the family together and now it had fallen apart. Six weeks of sessions with a psychologist helped me to understand what my feelings were about. She helped me to see what issues I needed to address and that had been plaguing me throughout my childhood and into adulthood.

In May 1985, I took off on a short but memorable trip to Tasmania. There, I hoped to connect with the one person who I felt was family, and who would understand my feelings; my surrogate aunty who had known me since I was seven years old when she had shared our family home. She had remained Mum's best friend and was now living in the Apple Isle, as it was commonly known, in reference to their apple industry. The first apple tree was planted by Captain William Bligh on Bruny Island, Tasmania in 1788.[8]

It was wonderful to see my aunty again and it was through her that I met two fascinating women. The first lady was working with Bach flower remedies in Huonville. The drive up a mountain to meet this homeopath was quite mystical. After we chatted, she made a tincture for me from the flowers that she grew in her garden. I took it each day and felt that it helped me gain clarity on what to do next. The inventor of these remedies, Dr Bach, I would later learn, believed in a truly holistic form of emotional healing and his remedies aim to assist the body in healing itself by providing:

> A positive emotional state that is conducive to the restoration of a healthy equilibrium and by acting to catalyze an individual's own internal resources for maintaining balance.[9]

The other lady I met was working with horses, using a form of energy healing from Japan. What amazed me most was that this woman was also treating a man, a farmer who she was helping by using this unusual form of healing. The farmer had rheumatoid arthritis. I was curious and wondered what he must be feeling, in so much pain, and with his body deformed and struggling to move. I watched as he received this healing energy and was impressed by how much it helped to reduce his pain. I asked the lady to lay her healing hands on me. I was so interested in this energy that was coming from her hands that I left there determined to find out where I could learn to do this healing myself.

I feel I have to explain why I was so open to this new idea of healing energy, which you could not see, and which was beyond the physical. Not since Edgar Cayce (1877-1945), the Sleeping Prophet, had anyone diagnosed illness in the body through channelling their energy into a person and going into a deep, sleep-like state or trance. Cayce would prescribe what the person needed to do to heal, which included a range of different modalities. I had several of his books at home. These healing modalities were so new to us in the West whereas Qi Gong and Acupuncture have been practised in the East and Meditation practised in India have all been around for thousands of years.

I returned home to Melbourne and was overjoyed to be back after so many years away, even though my immediate family were all living interstate. I was looking forward to reconnecting with old friends, hoping for a more stable lifestyle. I had decided that I wanted to live on my own. I found a cute little flat across from the beach in Elwood, which was an easy drive to work. I forgot about the healer in Tasmania, and all I could remember was that it was a form of Japanese healing energy.

Now happily employed as a casual in the X-ray department of a public hospital, I soon got promoted to what was called a floater. This meant going to different wards, collecting X-rays, and setting up rooms for the clinics. But it was so much more than that, and I loved it. Finally, I was happy and, life for me felt perfect.

My new boss took a chance on me and he offered me a full-time position. I enjoyed my work and my co-workers were lovely. I felt I had hit the jackpot. I had a fantastic job, a tremendous social life reconnecting with old friends, and a new, great little flat opposite the beach.

Unfortunately, life had other ideas. Since my promotion to full-time work, I initially thought that the aches and pains I was experiencing were due to the extra workload. Lifting heavy files of X-rays, unfortunately, became too much for me. My body felt sore and tired all the time and this was making me feel exhausted. Everything was such an effort. It was frustrating not knowing why.

Unknown to me, while working at the hospital, I had contracted two viruses—one was called Epstein-Barr virus (EBV) and the other was called Cytomegalovirus (CMV) infections. EBV is more commonly called Mono, "the kissing disease", or glandular fever, and its symptoms include fatigue, fever, lack of appetite, a rash, sore throat, swollen glands, and weakness. I learned that Cytomegalovirus is often caught while working in hospitals, and there is no preventative vaccine. While adults often have no symptoms of Cytomegalovirus, it can present like glandular fever with a fever, sore throat, swollen glands, and a sore abdomen. In hindsight, I think that it was contracting those two viruses together that created so much stress on my system. That, and the fact that I didn't want to stop working.

My local general practitioner had thought I was merely having a lot of sore throat issues, and so he did not test me for anything, and I carried on as best I could.

The day came, however, when I felt I was letting my new employer and the girls I worked with down so, rather than battling on any longer with the pain and tiredness, I quit my treasured job, and started looking for another. After all, I had always found work easily.

I had worked in so many different roles that I had learned it was easy to find work if you were versatile and willing to try your hand at anything. Constantly on the move, travelling both interstate and overseas, I had never stayed with the same company for more than twelve months. Basically, I was an employer's nightmare.

My gypsy lifestyle was entrenched early on. After attending twelve different schools, and then leaving school at the age of fifteen, I had lost my footing with school learning. We had little money growing up, and my parents moved for work often, so I had grown used to never staying in one place for too long. I became a life learner instead. By 1986, I counted thirty-eight jobs in total. I had been a fast-food cook in the Northern Territory, a reservations clerk in Sydney, and a cocktail mixer in Melbourne, to name a few. Although I had lost focus on school-based learning, working had brought me into contact with some amazing people and experiences.

I was only in my new position as a receptionist with a large company for a matter of weeks, though, when my whole system shut down completely.

It started in my hands. I found that I had no strength in my fingers to press the buttons needed to transfer calls. As hard as I pressed, I could not get any connections through. Frustrated, I had no idea what was going on. Understandably, my new workmates thought that I was just useless. *Let's face it,* I thought, *I pretty much am.* I was there to push buttons, and my fingers were having none of it.

Soon, I could feel no strength at all in my fingers or hands. It was so confusing. My body went progressively downhill from there. My fingers and hands were stiffening and locking up and, the day came when only a month in, I quit the receptionist position, and went for tests to find out what was going on with my body.

I was diagnosed with rheumatoid arthritis, a chronic inflammatory condition. This was the very disease I had been so curious about when I was staying in Tasmania. Here I was, a year later, learning firsthand what it was like to endure significant pain throughout my body, similar to the pain that farmer must have been going through. It was like alchemy. I had got my wish, my understanding of his situation. *Curiosity sometimes does kill the cat.*

I was set on a regimen of potent anti-inflammatories and was also put in touch with a pain clinic to help with my recovery, and to monitor my symptoms. The easy-going and caring clinic staff provided various techniques, gadgets, and tools to help me get through my day. Aids helped me to open jars, pull on my socks, and, eventually, a cane helped me to balance when walking. My exciting, full, and happy life had turned around and, suddenly, in the eyes of the Australian government, I had become an 87% disabled pensioner.

Chapter 4

The Medical Merry-Go-Round

In a dark time, the eye begins to see.
—*Theodore Roethke*[10]

When I reflect on my initial symptoms, my local GP had not followed through with enough tests. While working in the X-ray department at the hospital, I was a regular patient at my doctor's clinic, suffering recurring sore throats and constant fatigue, yet my GP did not dig deeper. I kept going as best I could. I had placed such stress on my body that my auto-immune system shut down.

In the local paper, I found a prominent clairvoyant. Desperate to find out what was going on with my body, I decided to pay her a visit. She told me that she could visualise me becoming healed. She said she could see me running up the aisles, it was like having a "hallelujah!" Faith healing. While the clairvoyant couldn't quite see how I would be healed, she knew that it would happen, and that all would be well. In the end, she was right. Unfortunately, my healing was still a way into the future. For now, life had other plans, and after giving up my treasured position at the hospital and then quitting my receptionist job, my lifestyle changed dramatically.

For the next three years, I became a disabled pensioner, living on a government invalid handout, and leading a life of restriction and pain.

Being told that I had rheumatoid arthritis was quite a surprise. I was young and felt that, at thirty, arthritis was an older person's disease. Yet, here I was with a walking cane, and hands that looked like they belonged to a senior citizen. I was confused as to how I had found myself in this position.

As author Kelly Noonan Gores wrote in her book *Heal* (2019):

> When a person shows up at a doctor's office and they receive a diagnosis of rheumatoid arthritis or MS or cancer or diabetes, once they hear that diagnosis, the common emotions they experience are either fear or sadness. They can think positively all they want. They can say, "I'm going to overcome this condition," but if they are feeling fear, that thought never makes it past the brain stem into the body because it's not in alignment with the body's emotional state. They need to become aware of where their thoughts are spiralling and bring them back to gratitude.[11]

Mostly, I had the right attitude about it all. Concentrating on healing my ill health became my new style of social life, and I learned about different and natural modalities, which are still my passion today.

Talking to a close friend recently, I asked her about what she remembered of me then. She said that I kept my pain and physical restrictions well hidden. She remembers that I still had fun, and that I was there for my friends. So, it seems I was not a complainer … except to my mum, at times.

Mum became my lifeline. Even though she was living umpteen thousand miles away in Katherine in the Northern

Territory, I called every week to let her know how I was coping. Mum has since told me that I had always kept things light or made a joke about my health issues. Part of my Pollyanna personality is that I can always find someone worse off and, for me, I think that is what helped me deal with what was happening. It's like I didn't want my physical restrictions and pain to define me as a person. Yet, here I was, classified an invalid. I remember a slogan that was popular on T-Shirts back then. It pictured a group of turkeys saying, *Don't let the Turkeys get you down.*[12] I resonated with that slogan. I loved it.

*

I soon discovered that I was wrongly diagnosed with having RA, or rheumatoid arthritis. The heavy-duty painkillers and anti-inflammatories that I was prescribed for RA were playing havoc with my stomach. I told a friend, and she suggested I see a naturopath.

This naturopath provided a shocking revelation. She told me that I didn't have RA, but that I had polyarthralgia. I was over the moon! The naturopath confirmed that I had contracted polyarthralgia due to my immune system shutting down after contracting both Epstein Barr virus and Cytomegalovirus.

As is typical with polyarthralgia, I found myself suffering from extensive joint pain in my hands and other parts of the body which is what lead to the initial misdiagnoses of rheumatoid arthritis. While polyarthralgia is more common among women, my case was unusual as I was so young, and the onset of this condition is usually associated with the elderly. Early on-set poly-arthralgia is apparently often caused by a virus. This was most definitely an influencing factor for me, as I suffered recurring bouts of illness ensuring that I was the perfect candidate for this debilitating condition.

The naturopath gave me some homeopathic medicines to treat the polyarthralgia, replacing the heavy-duty painkillers I had been prescribed.

Chapter 5

Give Up, Give In, or Give it Your All

In the middle of every difficulty lies opportunity.
—Albert Einstein[13]

O nce I knew that my condition was polyarthralgia, I discovered that the main treatment involved providing relief from my symptoms, which also meant improving my quality of life. Since polyarthralgia involves swelling of multiple joints, a combined approach of medications and therapy was recommended as most effective. I was referred to a pain clinic and from there to a physiotherapist to learn stretching and strengthening exercises at a heated pool. It was called hydrotherapy. To begin with, it was difficult to move my inflamed fingers and hands. At first even the simplest of movements was not easy as my body was so stiff and my range of movement limited. Pushing through the intense pain and stiffness, I persevered with the exercises, and I also restricted my diet.

After I'd been attending the pain clinic for a while, the staff recommended I see a psychiatrist to help me come to terms with the idea that my condition may not improve. So, I did. On the day of my appointment, I entered the room and sat down opposite a young male psychiatrist, waiting to hear what he had to say. I was hoping he would give me a positive outcome or a helpful suggestion as to what to continue doing.

Imagine my surprise and complete devastation when he bluntly said the words, 'You will be wheelchair-bound for life, and you need to come to terms with it.' He stood up and came over to where I was sitting. He then gave me what I am sure he thought was a consoling hug.

At that moment, the hug felt very condescending. After he had returned to his seat, I looked across at him and thought, *I am not going to accept what he was telling me. What does he know?* I remember thinking that this was not happening. *I will not be wheelchair-bound for life!* I think that psychiatrist's words were another catalyst in what I was to do next. Charleston Parker once said:

In life, you have three choices. Give up, give in, or give it your all. [14]

Luckily, the universe was placing all my ducks in a row. I had always been a doer, and I had lived life at a fast pace. Having attended twelve different schools there was hardly a sport that I had not tried, ranging from golf to horse riding. As a short, slim fifteen-year-old, I had worked at a local horse ranch and owned a tall fifteen-and-a-half hands ex-trotter who was way too much for me to handle. Brigadoon had bucked me off his back more times than I cared to remember, yet I continued to get right back on and ride again. Determination was part of my *modus operandi*, and that extended to skiing, ice skating, ten-pin bowling, roller skating, archery, and numerous other high energy sports. I had taken on thirty-eight different jobs by the time I was thirty years old, so I was a Jill of all trades, unafraid of new beginnings. I had lived in three different countries and four different states of Australia, so I loved being on the move. This confinement wasn't for me any longer.

Chapter 6

Magical Discoveries

You are capable of more than you know.
—*Glinda, the Good Witch from the Wizard of Oz*[15]

While I was with the pain clinic, a friend, Derek when he had some spare time from work and was feeling restless, acted as my driver, helping me seek out ways to reduce my symptoms. We had met at a local pub when his friend and my girlfriend started dating. I was not to know it then, but he was to also introduce me to my husband.

Floatation tanks were all the buzz and sessions there, along with hydrotherapy, soothed my joints. When I first started treatment, I must have looked like the Tin Man from *The Wizard of Oz,* or perhaps a robot that you see in popular science fiction movies—with fixed and rigid joints. I recall my absolute determination to get those 'joints' moving during hydrotherapy class with my physiotherapist. Standing in the warm, soothing water, after some sessions, I was able to move my shoulders and bring my elbows together, a considerable achievement. Running my stiffened fingers through the water, I pushed as hard as I could to regain my ability to curl my hands into fists.

I then discovered acupuncture, a great treatment that improved my range of movement and relieved the pain. Yoga too, was helping with my headspace. Practising all these modalities together, I felt I was taking charge of my health. It was great to know that I was no longer relying on NSAIDs (Non-Steroidal Anti-Inflammatory) pills to manage my symptoms, and I was feeling freer in my movements from each day to the next.

Floatation Tanks

I was terrified of floatation tanks at first. I am very claustrophobic. Just the thought of being enclosed in a tank of water with no one close by was something I wasn't looking forward to doing. I had to leave the lid open, which doesn't heighten the experience, but for me, it would do.

I was getting the benefit of relaxing my sore and swollen joints in the salt water and then, after a couple of sessions, I learnt to trust that I wasn't going to sink and drown or whatever crazy thought I had at the time. I was able to let go and float around in the dark and just drift off, listening to music and really enjoying my time in the tank. The bonus was that my painful joints felt so relieved after those sessions, and my mind was at peace. The salt that gets clogged in your ears was not so great, but that was a minor hassle. I recommend floatation tanks if you have painful joints.

All these therapies I continued to practise over the next couple of years. The yoga, floatation tanks, hydrotherapy, physiotherapy, and acupuncture, combined with the vitamins and dietary changes I had made, helped me to recover, but I was yet to discover the therapy that would prove to be the icing on the cake.

I also believed that I was ready—the timing was right. I was ready to leave the constrictions of the pain clinic behind, ready to leave their diagnosis behind, and ready to find my own way to healing.

Reiki 1

"Miracles happen every day with Reiki"—wrote Sue for the *John Harvey Gray Centre for Reiki,* in June 2014.[16] I was to learn how very true this is. Back in the 1980s, Reiki was largely unheard of in Australia, and spiritual healing or the laying on of hands was mainly conducted in spiritual churches.

It is widely agreed that the Reiki method of healing originated in 1922, introduced by the Japanese spiritual leader, Dr Mikao Usi. He is said to have begun teaching others after a serious earthquake hit Japan and he felt the need to spread his knowledge.[17]

Reiki can be described as a form of energy healing. The palms of the healer are placed lightly on the patient's body, or hover just above it. It creates a movement of energy through the body with the intention of healing both physical and emotional ailments. It can create a deeply relaxed state where the patient may find that it releases blocked and suppressed feelings, it can reduce stress and promote creativity. It is also known to be balance energies and strengthen the immune system, speed the healing processes in the body and can reduce pain.

*

Three years after starting my life of pain and deformity, I began to experience energy healing in the form of Reiki. My friend Sybil, who had introduced me to the joy of cross-country snow skiing and who had very arthritic hands herself, told me about this woman she had been to see, and that her Reiki sessions would help me. I called and made an appointment with this practitioner and was amazed by what happened.

Here I was lying on the practitioner's massage table having my healing. I had no idea what was happening, as my eyes were closed, and for those of you who have not had some form of this healing, sometimes a tissue or an eye mask is placed over your eyes.

I was lying there feeling calm and peaceful when, all of a sudden, I felt my body shift and take on a different shape. I felt heavier in my body. It seems I was male, and my head felt heavy. It felt like I was wearing some form of a helmet. It appeared to be made of a glass of some sort, and then I saw colours, all the rainbow colours, in my head. I tried to speak, and my voice came out gruff and low. The woman went rushing from the room. She brought back a friend to witness what I was going through.

It seemed my head covering was crystal. I had regressed back to a past life, to when I was a priest of an ancient city, working with crystals. This, funnily enough, didn't surprise me. From when I was very young, I had always collected semiprecious stones and rocks.

I remember being exhausted after this session, but also excited by what had happened. I had gone straight into a past life regression and, even though I am quite a spiritual person, this didn't faze me too much, it was still a different state of being over which I had no control. It was all so very new to me, and that first session was quite profound. Soon I was back seeing this woman for two more sessions of that energy healing. After only my third session, I was able to throw away the cane I used for walking. My new neighbours couldn't believe the changes in me. Although I was not exactly striding up the stairs with ease, I could now move with comparative agility.

By this time, I had moved to a new house, and my new abode was up flights of stairs opposite Luna Park. The noise and the screams from the patrons on the rollercoaster and the lights were a perfect change after the quietness of my previous home. I began to feel connected again—to people, to life, and to living. Not only did I love the location, but my neighbours, David and his friend, Clare, and a couple of others who lived on the block, looked out for me, and we became good friends.

Due to my condition, my diet over the previous three years had changed drastically. Living on a pension too, I only had so much to spend after paying rent. I remember making up pumpkin soup for fifty cents once and eating only that for three days running. One Christmas during this time, my lovely, thoughtful uncle, drove an hour each way to deliver me a basket of chicken and vegetables.

Soon, Reiki became an essential part of my routine, and my life took a fantastic turnaround. After only a few weeks of regular Reiki sessions, my body began on a path towards ultimate healing. I started to see that I would no longer live with limitations or purely exist on an invalid pension.

After those initial sessions, that was it—I wanted my life back. I could see light at the end of the tunnel, and I wanted to do a course on Reiki healing. As I have no diaries from either 1986 or 1987, the only evidence of my healing journey is a date written on a calendar that reads, 'Reiki 1 $125.' It was August 1988 and a Friday evening start. That night, I was lucky enough to meet a lovely couple, Dianne, and Jeff, who took me under their wing.

The problem I had with my hands during the Reiki positions was holding them so that they lay flat on my body. My fingers were bent out of shape, so getting them to lie flat was hard and, at times, I needed help from the class assistants to flatten my hands down into position. But I managed and even today, thirty years later, I remember that feeling of achievement.

I have since read that the first Reiki attunement can provide an extremely powerful opening for a student who is ready for such an opening[18]. This is rare, though. Most people, as author Amy Rowland suggests, have some mild sensation of energy flowing through their hands or in their heads, and yet others feel no difference at all. In *The Complete Book of Traditional Reiki*, Rowland explains that this is fine, that the energy becomes more apparent with each subsequent attunement, and that the sensations experienced are not of the practitioner's choosing, but are expressions of the healing energy flowing through the practitioner to meet the needs of the client.

After completing Reiki 1, and on such a high from my success, I visited arthritis centres and offered my services to the ladies there to help them get movement back into their hands. Sadly, they looked at me as if I was crazy. Once again, as this was thirty years ago, Reiki was not well known, and they possibly didn't believe me because, my hands had started to heal.

It's funny—the joy you get from certain things after not having them for a while. Luckily, both my hands and feet reverted to almost what they were before, but my handwriting was never the same. I consider this such a small price to pay.

Recently, I found a twenty-month weekly schedule that I had started to write from August 1988. There, in October, it lists me travelling again, as you do when you are a genuine nomad. Once again, I was cashed up, fitter and healthier, and taking a sleeper train north to Queensland to catch up with family and go to see World Expo '88 in Brisbane. At that stage, I was sharing my Reiki healing for barter—a Reiki session in exchange for a bed for the night, or a coffee, at times. This system proved to be good practice for me, while it also spread news of my experience up and down the Queensland coast.

Returning from my trip, I had an idea of possibly earning money by doing healings. *Could this be my new career? Perhaps, I could even work with animals?*

Dianne from the Reiki 1 course and I had grown close, and her relationship with Jeff had begun to fall apart, so we talked about moving in together to share a house. I found us a big, four-bedroom house in Caulfield, Victoria. Soon after, Dianne had reconnected with her previous love and moved in with him. I was happy for them, they eventually got married, but I was now on the lookout for new housemates.

I felt that I could become a Reiki practitioner and help others. I bought a massage table, and another friend of mine made up business cards for me to hand out. I was ready, or so I thought. I had moved into my share house, and I took my new flatmate along with me to a greyhound racing-track. I thought I would begin by working with animals first, then people. I took some business cards, and a great sense of hope. Waiting until the race was run, I approached the owners of the losing greyhounds and offered my services. I tried to explain how Reiki energy would help their dogs. 'It could possibly make him stronger and help him to win,' I said. Funnily enough, my pitch didn't go over too well. *What on earth was I thinking!* I am not sure whether I thought I could give the greyhounds a boost of energy or help heal their muscles from the race. Whatever my plan was at the time, it backfired. Thinking back, a racetrack probably wasn't the best place to try out my animal healing skills. Perhaps a veterinarian practice might have been a better venue and target audience, but I think it was probably still early for me too.

Reiki 2

I signed up for the Reiki 2 course in February 1989. Unfortunately, I was hospitalised on the Saturday before I was meant to start. That day, I had been ill, throwing up bile, so my lovely neighbour took me to the Prince Alfred Hospital.

The surgeon told me that I had adhesions from my previous stomach surgery, and that I needed to be opened up again, so that they could clear away the tissue. The positives from this surgery included a much slimmer scar running from my belly button down the length of my stomach, after my original abdominal surgery. My surgery took place on Sunday, and my Reiki workshop was to begin the following Friday.

I contacted the Reiki 2 course trainers. I was sure that my pain levels could drop or diminish significantly due to all the energy I would be transferring during the course. So, signing myself out of the hospital shortly after having surgery I felt, was a smart thing to do. I discharged myself the day before Reiki 2 began. As the saying goes, "Whatever you give your attention to, be it positive or negative, is what feeds you." I was eating positivity for breakfast, lunch, and dinner back then.

Reiki 2, for me, proved to be another of my life's highlights. The workshops were held each Friday evening and all weekend, and I couldn't wait for the next attunement. I loved Reiki. I became ready, not only to share Reiki, but to share love also. I began to view Reiki energy as like a "hug drug".

My Reiki course was held in South Yarra. I was so determined to attend it to the end, which I was able to do and I enjoyed the greatest healing. I found that, while I was learning, I was also receiving. It is a win-win! You are being healed while healing. You also learned distance healing. As my family were living interstate, I wanted to help them, if they needed me.

*

Over the years, I have met many women and some men who have finished the Reiki course, and they are often so excited that they want to share it with others. It is great to see. During our training, the hundredth monkey effect was used as an understanding. In his book, *The Hundredth Monkey*, Ken Keyes explains how a new behaviour or idea can spread rapidly from one group to all groups— it's about societal change. The story goes that back in Japan in the 1950s, scientists were giving monkeys sweet potatoes, which they liked: well, who wouldn't? I love them. However, the scientists were dropping the potatoes in the sand, which didn't appeal to the monkeys' taste buds. After a while, one female monkey—it seems to always take a clever woman—started washing her sweet potatoes in a nearby stream. She then taught her technique to the other monkeys in her group. Soon, all the monkeys were washing their sweet potatoes. What was more unusual was that monkeys on different islands also began to do the same. They say that the hundredth monkey effect is about how awareness can be communicated from mind to mind. The group needs to comprise of a certain size, but there is no exact number.[19]

*

After completing Reiki 2, spiritual healing became such a passion for me that I turned into a workshop junkie, adding many other strings to my bow. I felt the need to know more about different healing modalities. Over the years, I learnt: Touch for Health

Kinesiology and Kinergy; Spiritual Healing, with someone who is quite well known; Animal Dreaming with Scott Alexander King, which was a lot of fun, and Crystal Bed Healing. This one was an absolute must as I had always been surrounded by crystals from a young age. I also went on to learn Seichim which is a female form of Reiki, The Horstmann Technique, and Pellowah. I loved finding out more about myself which I did with Face Reading with Hermann Muller, and there have been a few more. Each one of these modalities I have found enlightening and inspiring. I have loved them all and gained such knowledge. Each, in their own way, has added to my life, and helped me heal. However, I have always returned to my first love, which is Reiki.

My lovely neighbour, David, the one who had helped me reach hospital for my stomach operation, used to tell me that all the spiritual healing I was learning about was rubbish. He repeatedly told me that he didn't believe in it. However, the day came when David had a nasty headache. He came knocking on my door and asked if I could place my hands on his head to soothe the pain. I did, and he happily enjoyed the healing benefits.

It wasn't until I had completed the Reiki 2 course that I felt I could start doing some form of work again. Taking on another's pain is not something you do with Reiki but, with me, that is just how it happens, at times. When a client is dealing with specific emotional issues, I feel like the Reiki is also clearing my own. Other times, the energy flows through smoothly. I began to learn that every client and every experience is different. At times, cold energy has come through, freezing my hands up to the elbow. At other times, the energy runs very hot. And people's bodies react differently. Sometimes, they exhibit little twitches, flicks, or muscle spasms, while others, like me, see different colours. I have learned that we all get what is needed at that particular time.

When working with one memorable client, my hands felt like they had dropped inside their body. I felt as if I was holding their organs in my hands. At other times, a stream of information has come through for me to share with the person and, for others still, their treatment has meant a restful sleep.

Along the way, many people have told me that they don't believe in Reiki or spiritual healing. 'It's all woo-woo,' they say, while others became excited when I discussed with them this new energy. Over the years, I have learned that we are all individuals. What one person will gravitate to, is different for another.

Reiki can now be taught on DVD—no longer do you need someone to guide you through it. However, I believe that many people enjoy the process of experiencing the energy and learning Reiki together. I believe it's a tribal thing. Also, I think that a shared experience is worthwhile because each person has a different response to the healing energy, and it is helpful to understand some of the unusual sensations that might happen for others.

Reiki allowed me to discover that, when a group of people came together, miracles happened, or at least the synchronicity for healing occurred. We helped one another, and shared brilliant experiences. More than that, I felt that I had finally found my tribe.

Sadly, by this time my dear friend, Derek, who had acted as my personal chauffeur during my time on the invalid pension, was leaving and heading back to his hometown. He had fronted up when he wasn't working, and he had been a great help to me. He enjoyed finding out about all these healing modalities, but he was not interested in doing any of them for himself. I have come to understand that people come into our lives to help us on our path. His parting gift was bringing his friend, now my husband and myself together on a blind date. The rest, as they say, is history.

Chapter 7

Find Your Healing

We can all change our outlook, our thought processes. Famed meditation and Japanese yoga instructor, H E Davey once said:

> The mind moves the body, and the body follows the mind. Logically then, negative thought patterns harm not only the mind but also the body.[20]

Through researching how to heal myself, not only did I discover many different alternative healing modalities for my body, I also challenged my mindset. I began to view the cause of my illness, and therefore its treatment, from a different perspective. Ultimately, this combined learning led to my recovery.

Naturopathy, including Bach's Flower Remedies

As far as alternative therapies go, most people are familiar with the term Naturopathy. As the name would suggest, Naturopaths are trained to use the healing power of nature and apply a combination of therapies to help their patients. They look at preventing an illness and believe in an approach that is a combination of both art and science ...

Initially, I would see my GP and then proceed to a Naturopath for my supplements and vitamins; I feel that this helped me in my wellbeing.

Naturopathy[21] uses a holistic approach for people's health and can include herbal and nutritional medicines, as well as massages, acupuncture, and other dietary or lifestyle changes or recommendations.

My first introduction to homeopathy, although I was unaware at the time, was that trip to Tasmania in the mid-1980s when I met the old European lady using Bach's Flower Remedies to heal others. I later discovered that Dr Edward Bach believed that:

> … the presence of an illness always implies conflict between what the person wants and the life plan of the person's soul. [22]

The mention of a person's soul and its impact on a person's health resonated with me. I loved reading about Bach's view on illness being a result of a person's inability or refusal to listen to what their soul truly wanted. Additionally, he believed that "illness is a method of bringing us back to the path of understanding". *I loved reading this.*

Energy Work

Meditation and Your Mind Power
In his book, *When the Body Says No. The Cost of Hidden Stress* (2019), Gabor Maté shares that:

> … a mind-body perspective may help those afflicted with ALS (Amyotrophic Lateral Sclerosis, also known as motor neurone disease) who are willing to look at some very painful realities fully and unflinchingly.[23]

In rare instances, Maté states that people do seem to get over symptoms diagnosed as ALS. Maté quotes the case reported by Dr Christiane Northrup of Dana Johnson, a registered nurse, who recovered from Lou Gehrig's disease by learning to respect all aspects of her body.

In Dana's story, she outlines her daily ritual of sitting in front of a mirror in her wheelchair and spending 15 minutes on a part of her body to love. While doing this she also wrote in her journal. She wrote of her life focused on sacrificing to help others. Documenting this helped her to understand that this behaviour was detrimental to her own health and may have contributed to her illness. Finally taking the time to assess her life during this dark and painful time, she began to love herself, and according to Dr Northrup, her friend Dana healed through a conscious daily practice of emotional self-inventory and of self-love that, little by little, unfroze each part of her body.

Maté also goes on to state in a chapter of *When the Body Says No. The Cost of Hidden Stress* (2019) called, The Power of Negative Thinking:

> The potential for wholeness for health resides in all of us as does the potential for illness and disharmony. Disease is disharmony. More accurately, it is an expression of an internal disharmony.[23]
>
> The first step in retracing our way to health is to abandon our attachment to what is called positive thinking. "I have always been a positive thinker," one man in his late 40s told me. "I have never given in to pessimistic thoughts. Why should I get cancer?"
>
> As an antidote to terminal optimism, I have recommended the power of negative thinking. Tongue in cheek, of course. What I really believe in is the power of thinking. As soon as we can't qualify the word thinking with the attitude adjective positive, we exclude those parts

of reality that strike us as "negative". That is how most people who espouse positive thinking seem to operate. Genuine positive thinking begins by including all our reality. It is guided by the confidence that we can trust ourselves to face the full truth, whatever that full truth may turn out to be.

Nowadays when I talk with my mum on the phone, I don't gloss over things that might be making me angry or sad and Mum does the same. We both say at the end of our conversation that it is good to get it out of our system, so that we are not carrying the negativity in our bodies.

Tapping

Tapping, or EFT (Emotional Freedom Techniques) Tapping is seen as an alternative to acupuncture and involves the physical tapping of a series of acupressure points on the body that can help the patient access their meridian energies while focussing on a particular emotional or physical issue. It is a treatment that is easy to learn and to self-administer and can help with issues ranging from anxiety through to pain management.

*

Nicolas Ortner is CEO of The Tapping Solution. In his book, *The Tapping Solution for Pain Relief* (2015), Ortner explains that:

> Some experts believe that the nature and timing of the specific neuroplastic changes in the brain that happen after an injury may affect where, and for how long, you experience pain from that injury.[24]

Ortner also states that:

Research has clearly shown that adverse experiences, unresolved emotions, and events from childhood don't just make a mark on our memories; they have a lasting impact on the body.

Ortner quotes the Adverse Childhood Experiences (ACE Study), a research project funded by Kaiser Permanente and the Centers for Disease Control in the US, which followed 17 000 participants and found that: " … unresolved childhood trauma has profound effects on the body well into adulthood." The study confirmed direct correlations between childhood trauma and cancer, heart disease, diabetes, stroke, high blood pressure, bone fracture, depression, and drug use.[25]

Recently, I was tapping along with Brad Yates of *Tap with Brad;*[26] "Being Consistent" was the topic of the day. *Wow! Talk about timing.* I tapped away my struggle of years of being inconsistent and tapped how it would be beneficial to be consistent daily, for my health. I tapped about consistently doing evening meditations as I went to sleep, and a two-minute Harvard or Wonder Woman pose each morning. I knew that many healing benefits would come my way if I was more consistent. I am still working on it!

Kinesiology

The very first time that I had a session with a kinesiologist, I thought it was odd, even after my first Reiki session. The woman was doing weird facial expressions, and her mouth was opening and closing, a bit like a goldfish. At the same time, she was kicking one of her legs out to the side at 45-degree angle. I was thinking, *What is going on?* It was comical. It turned out to be a fantastic session, however, and I went on to learn different kinds of kinesiology for myself and that there are different ways of muscle testing your body for information and healing.

Kinesiology is a form of muscle testing and is used to detect physical and emotional imbalances in the body. Kinesiology finds and releases tension in the body and mind. It can also help with dietary issues. It helped me find a sugar imbalance, helped to find allergies, and candida in my body that were creating many health issues. Donna Eden, who was diagnosed with MS in her teens, teaches what she calls, Energy Kinesiology.

Naturopathy uses herbal treatments, as well as homeopathy and diet, while looking at the root cause of the illness. Kinesiology, by contrast, tests the muscles in your body, which can be holding onto tension in both the body and mind. Kinesiology can find dietary intolerances by holding specific foods to the body, testing to see how the body is made stronger or weaker.

Kinesiology has also proven useful in treating learning problems, which is great for kids.

Top tennis player, Novak Djokovic, apparently credits Kinesiology with helping him find a gluten intolerance.

Qi Gong

I had enjoyed yoga, but now wanted to try Qi Gong. A few years after finding Reiki, I joined a large group, sitting on plastic chairs in a park in South Yarra. We listened to a man named Jack Lim as he explained about the energy of Qi Gong, whereupon he gave a demonstration. He lifted his hand and said that he would direct his energy to a woman sitting directly across from him, a good distance away. When he had finished, he asked what she had felt. She replied, 'Nothing.' This was because Jack had been a little off in his direction. I was sitting next to her and had been the receiver. My body had begun to slowly slide down off the chair, and I was struggling to stay upright. Luckily for me, Jack finished when he did, otherwise, I would have been laid out, splat on the ground. Of course,

I signed up straight away. *How good was this!* Another healing energy therapy to add. I was on a path to becoming an energy healing junkie.

Reiki

Reiki (pronounced ray-key) is a Japanese form of spiritual healing using universal life energy that is channelled through the practitioner to the recipient.[27] The contribution Reiki has made to my own healing has been enormous. For me it was a cornerstone to all of the other therapies that I undertook and still one that I use today. It keeps me balanced and I instinctively turn to it; it is part of who I am and how I interact with the world. Reiki's ability to align your own, or a patient's body, mind and spirit is part of what makes it such a powerful healing and gentle modality.

During a Reiki treatment, which would typically last for around an hour, the practitioner would address all of the organs in the body, holding their palms open just above you, or gently on you while you are seated or lying down, full clothed with your eyes closed and often covered. While experiences do vary, most people find it to be a very relaxing and soothing experience as the practitioner controls the energy flow around their body. Some experience warmth and tingling and as there is no pressure on the body, it is seen to be ideal for treating a range of conditions on a range of people from the very young to the elderly.

Reiki it is said, promotes natural self-healing, balances energies, strengthens the immune system, treats symptoms and causes of illness, relieves pain, clears toxins, and adapts to the natural needs of the receiver.

Please note that Reiki should never be used instead of medical treatment. It should be used as a complementary healing method.

You may also find that your hands turn on at different times, and you feel the flow of Reiki energy. This is something that happens to me to this day. You may also soon discover too that your ego and spirit can survive the scepticism of others. Reiki's healing energy is not affected by other opinions as I learnt from my lovely neighbour David.

*

One day, my hubby and I had taken our dog over to our closest dog park, and I had only just sat down on the bench when a gorgeous young golden retriever backed himself into my knees. I started slowly rubbing my hands over his back and down to his tail. He quite happily took it in, but I got a bit of a surprise. My husband who had let our dog off to have a run, came over to me.

'Lovely dog,' he said.

'Yes, he is,' I replied, 'but he's riddled with arthritis.'

Next minute, the dog's young owner came over. We told her that she had a beautiful dog.

'Yes,' she said, 'but he's not even a year old, and his body is full of arthritis.'

I felt so sad for that beautiful but happy dog, thinking of what he had to go through at such a young age.

These days, dogs, cats, and horses have acupuncture, chiropractic work, and energy work. I also know of or two practices here in Queensland who use Reiki energy.

Our two chows just love having acupuncture. Our lovely therapist, Karen, comes to our home and the boys get so excited to see her. Karen sits down in front of them and they push each other out of the way, no manners here, wanting their treatment. They push their butts up against her waiting for the needles to be inserted. One of the chows has hip dysplasia and the other has arthritis. Both are doing well.

*

It seems that my life journey of chronic illness was like a domino effect. One thing led to another, and then another, and so on. Environment, early emotional issues, and toxicity all had their part to play, and it was too much for this little body. Each time I tried one of these new healing modalities, I was so excited. They worked, and another issue was dealt with. I am not alone. It seems that many of our well-known stars of the screen use different healing modalities. Angelina Jolie, Kate Hudson, and Naomi Watts, are said to use Reiki healing. Miranda Kerr practises yoga, as do Eva Longoria and Charlize Theron.

Chapter 8

A Path Oft Travelled

... what is essential is invisible to the eye.
—Antoine de Saint-Exupéry[28]

It was 2017, and I was struggling with another illness that had been long-winded, not easy to diagnose, and needed extra help from the universe to address. After all the special diets, some starvation, and a multitude of vitamins, herbs, and minerals, I began to head back down the familiar path.

I returned to Reiki—to the most profound healing for me and my body, and to meditation for my brain. This, along with my new diet, means that I am happy to say I am doing well.

I want to share what I was going through and had gone through up to that time. I had received a diagnosis of MTHFR gene mutation, and food histamine intolerance. Genetic mutations come from your parents. There are two types of this gene mutation. I have the one which is to do with the body's ability to turn folic acid into folate. This genetic mutation may lead to high levels of an amino acid called homocysteine in the blood which can increase the risk of heart attacks, strokes, low levels of folate, and other vitamin deficiencies. Symptoms of this gene mutation may include, digestive issues, migraines, nerve pain, depression, anxiety, and chronic fatigue.

I have experienced some of these symptoms apart from depression and schizophrenia. But I now understand how anxiety can play havoc in everyday life. Luckily, the days of me double or triple checking the locks on the doors before leaving home have now abated after changing my diet.

Thankfully, issues caused by this genetic mutation can be minimised with the right diet, supplements, and lifestyle choices.

Anthony William, the Medical Medium, wrote about the MTHFR gene in his book, *Liver Rescue* (2018), in which he goes into about the role our liver has in our overall wellbeing and the impact of the MTHFR gene mutation. Another author is, Dr Ben Lynch, and his book *Dirty Genes* (2018), in which he talks about own his health issues and the impact of lifestyle, diet and mindset can affect genes and their ability to function. It is also encouraging to see the amount of information available online; the references section at the end of my book provides some suggested websites on this condition.

I found that the food I had been eating large amounts of: vinegars in salads with balsamic, especially, but also red wine, white, and apple cider vinegar, and roughly two avocados a week, a breakfast of raspberries and strawberries with yoghurt and a cup of green tea, or bone broth, leafy green baby spinach in all of my salads … sounds fairly healthy, you would think … lemons and limes from my fruit trees, and my favourite, red grapefruit—all of these foods had helped lead me to an overbalance or overflowing bucket of high histamines, which caused many strange things to happen in my body. I would be sitting at my desk and have a mini blackout. This happened not long after I was diagnosed.

My hubby and I had gone to Bali for a five-day holiday. Luckily, we were in our room at the time. I managed to stagger to the bed, and I had a blackout—a short loss of consciousness. My husband hadn't seen this happen to anyone before and, what horrified him most, was my face. It had puffed up so much that he didn't recognise me. The photo he took of me was a shock to us both. It was not so flattering!

In his book, *Medical Medium* (2015), Anthony William states that:

> There's a misconception that because fermented foods helped humans along for thousands of years, they have health benefits.[29]

Anthony William explains that these foods were about survival. They were "historical stopgaps" rather than a health aid. Anthony William clarifies that:

> The so-called probiotics in fermented foods are not life-giving. The bacteria in them thrive off the decay process—in other words, they thrive off death, not life.

When I read this, I wondered how it is that there aren't more of us out there with high histamine food problems. As he says, we need living foods in fruit and vegetables to thrive. They have a life force that the bacteria in fermented foods do not. He also advises that, if you're struggling with a health condition, though, yoghurt is not a positive food to consume; dairy feeds all manner of ills.[30]

Such bacteria from so many of these foods—foods that aren't alive—are useless to your gut. Anthony William also states that if you like fermented foods for their flavour (which I must admit I loved) and if fermented foods don't upset your stomach, then eat them. It seems that they just aren't as healthy for us as we thought and provide little benefit.

Here was I thinking that I was doing the right thing by eating in a healthy way, and I was making things so much worse for my poor stomach. Anthony William also talks about the different kinds of vinegar. While apple cider vinegar gets a better rap than all the others, I was taking it daily. Yet, with the issues that I have, this was a definite no-no, as the vinegar was irritating my gut. I have been off fermented foods and vinegar for more than eighteen months and, although I miss my yoghurts, even my coconut ones, and the tart taste of the vinegars in my food, I know that I need to get my gut into balance.

Dr Joseph Pizzorno has spent nearly fifty years exploring the connection between toxins and human health. In *The Toxin Solution* (2018), Dr Pizzorno says that the gut and the digestive tract are where detox must always start:

> If your gut is overflowing with toxins it can't process, it will pass it along to other areas of your body undermining those organs.[31]

There are a lot of great tips in his book. He says that:

> … if you use marijuana use the forms that are least toxic. It seems a lot of pesticides and herbicides can be used during their growing.[32]

This is something I never would have thought about!

Another interesting insight I learned from Dr Pizzorno is that, if your liver is not detoxing effectively, you will have a strong odour after eating asparagus, caffeine—even small amounts—will keep you awake at night, an intolerance to perfume, strong odours, and you will experience gut imbalance.

I learned too that high histamine foods include fermented kombucha, bone broth, and sauerkraut. According to Sydney nutritionist and skin expert Fiona Tuck, these foods may fuel outbreaks for histamine intolerance sufferers[33]. The condition is quite often confused with hay fever because it presents unexplainable allergy-type symptoms, but tests negative to allergies. Tuck states:

> Increased histamine may aggravate symptoms such as gastric stress, nausea, headaches, mood disorders, sinus problems, skin rashes, breathing difficulties, itching and burning eyes, and flushing of the skin.[34]

High histamine foods include fermented and aged foods, cheeses, citrus fruits, tomatoes, avocados, and chocolate. Sufferers should also avoid coffee, black and green tea, and alcohol as these inhibit the DAO enzyme that helps break down histamine. Instead, Tuck recommends eating antihistamine foods: watercress, onions, garlic, holy basil, thyme, nettle, peppermint, ginger and apples. Over the counter medications that may help alleviate symptoms include magnesium, quercetin, vitamin B6, and pancreatic enzymes. But she urges people not to self-diagnose.

Quite often, I was experiencing pins and needles in my hands and feet, feeling bloated, and I was experiencing vertigo, which is not pleasant. It seems that the MTHFR gene, and histamines are closely related. The Medical Medium, Anthony William, says that these symptoms are the result of "dirty blood". I have now started on a liver-cleansing diet to help cleanse my blood.

It's time to share some of the other health issues that I have been dealing with throughout my journey. My major source of pain is in my back. I have Scheuermann's kyphosis, a disease of the spine, which at times, has kept me locked in place, unable to move forwards or backwards, to turn left or right from my hips upward. I find sometimes I move like the Tin Man in the *Wizard of Oz … Not great if you are doing yoga that day!*

Fibromyalgia, which was diagnosed back when I was in my late twenties, was reconfirmed by a rheumatologist not so long ago. I can have years of it not affecting me, and then, back it comes, mainly brought on by the stressors of life at the time. I have been renovating a house for the past nine years, so there have been a few. I experience aching muscles and a lot of fatigue. It has been said that fibromyalgia is the disease of the overachiever as many sportspersons are confirmed sufferers.

I also have spinal stenosis in my L4 and L5 vertebrae, in the lower part of my spine. I also have the exotic sounding Cauda Equina syndrome (Latin: horse tail), which is a compression of the nerve roots at the end of your spine. It is called that because, on imaging, it resembles a horse's tail. *It really does!*

All these things combined can make life a little tricky at times, but not impossible. I find that if I don't give my focus to them, life is great. For the pain, back in the day, I used to be on heavy medication, which I stopped taking because of my gut problems. Then, I used alcohol, white wine mostly, for my pain relief, which was not good for my liver. Until I started a food diary, which was to try to discover was happening to my body again, I did not realise how much of a habit my two glasses of wine a night had become.

That self-medicating became greatly restricted once I found out that I now have a food histamine intolerance. I have regular acupuncture along with some kinesiology, I take my herbal supplements, use essential oils, and I treat myself with ten-minute Reiki sessions.

I discovered that my body had a strange reaction to folic acid. In my thirties, I had endured five rounds of IVF, but could not progress pregnancies past three months. I learned that the mutations to my MTHFR gene meant that folic acid was toxic to early pregnancy for me and would abort a foetus. Hospitals are now aware of this, and I have read that testing for the common versions or polymorphisms in the MTHFR gene is now available.

My mother once told me that I had a twin who died at birth. Mum believed that I was carrying the illnesses for two—not a good thing to have locked into your subconscious. I am still working on this area of my genetic makeup and past. Mum lost eight babies through miscarriage. This supports the defect in my MTHFR genetics, but many other factors also come into play for me. My mother's grandmother also lost eight children of the thirteen she gave birth to. Knowing that folic acid was not a good thing for me to take while trying to fall pregnant would have helped when I was wanting to have children.

Many blogs and books now help to explain food intolerances. Each time I had thought that my health issues had led me onto a better way of eating. When I was diagnosed over twelve years ago with coeliac disease, I removed gluten and some grains from my diet. When I developed issues with eating dairy—even though I adore cheese and chocolate and let's not leave out ice cream—my skin seemed to benefit, and my dermatitis cleared up. I removed so many problems by changing my diet. With this latest food/histamine allergy or intolerance, I changed my diet again, hoping to help my liver. I feel that all these changes to my diet have been for the better. I have learned that your body does speak to you—we have to find the correct translator to help us navigate the messages.

What I have also learnt from my food intolerances is that there is a definite gut-brain connection. The anxiety that I was experiencing for over a year or more where I would continuously check our doors to make sure they were locked, including at times, returning home after leaving the house to check them again, disappeared once I cut high histamine food from my diet. The frustration of doing this had been driving me crazy. I knew it was irrational, yet I couldn't stop myself. *How many other things can be helped by a change of diet?* I wonder.

While I was finding out what foods I was reacting to, I came across a website called, *Healing Histamine*.[35] Yasmina was born in a war-torn country which she had left at a young age. She also had the similar issue as me of moving schools every six to twelve months. Yasmina was dealing with food issues while working as a journalist for both CNN and the BBC covering war zones. She devoted her skills to researching and writing about histamine and I found her site to be invaluable.

A well-known chef here in Australia, Pete Evans, who I have followed for years, watching his shows on TV, advocates the benefits of a Paleo diet. I am now on this paleo diet and it is the one, and with Yasmina's information I believe, that is right for me.

'Paleo is very beneficial,' Evans previously told Daily Mail Australia.

'It's a way of returning to a far more natural way of eating and a way of using the foods you eat to drive optimal health and balance in your body.'

'By ditching refined carbohydrates and sugars and replacing them with moderate amounts of protein, good-quality fats and lots of nutrient-dense vegetables, you'll have energy to burn.'[36]

Another chef, Lee Holmes is a nutritionist and the author of *Supercharge Your Life: How to put real food at the heart of everything* (2019). Holmes advises us to:

Eat foods for the sake of genuine enjoyment rather than for some other agenda, such as a diet or a particular health outcome.[37]

When reading this, I thought, *Yes! I have always loved food.* I can cook up a storm, but when I started getting allergies— over the past twelve or so years—first with wheat and gluten, then with dairy and now with high histamine foods—each time, it was a huge disappointment. Recently, I found myself telling someone about my favourite foods, and how excited I am eating from my limited food base. It's a different style of eating; fresh foods and less complicated, yet I can still be creative.

Lee Holmes writes in *Supercharge Your Life* (2019), that in the last decade, science has been unveiling the fascinating connection between our mind and body. Previously, we thought there were narrow cause and effect links between the food we ate and health outcomes, but we are now learning that our minds and thinking play an immensely important role in the way our physical body functions. These breakthroughs have come through the study of epigenetics and how our genes are expressed and learning about the neuroplasticity of the microbiome in the brain.

Tapping on dental problems

The first time I used tapping was after being diagnosed with a food allergy, so this was over ten years ago. I really love my food, so I wanted to be able to eat wheat again. I was desperate for my pasta and pizzas and, at that time, having a food allergy wasn't as easy to cope with as it is today. I was tapping on my face so hard, it's a wonder I didn't leave bruises. I wasn't consistent with it, though—I didn't tap away daily, and I stopped after I found that not eating wheat helped ease a lot of pain in my body. Becoming gluten-free also helped with some skin problems and, in the end, it was an easy change.

I'm not sure I believed it could really help me at the time, but I later read about a guy who had cured himself of MS (multiple sclerosis) through tapping. I tried tapping again, but this time it was for emotional issues, and now I do very gentle tapping—light and easy, not a frantic whack! whack! whack! at my face.

Mum had a stressful time when a large molar was removed at a dental visit. It had taken over an hour for the tooth to come out, and Mum was told that she needed to come back the following week to remove another molar. Unhappy about this, Mum asked me what she should do. Mum wanted to avoid the same thing happening as having dental work is not her favourite thing.

I had just started EFT tapping, so suggested that Mum try it every day that week, focusing on the upcoming dental work being a more positive experience. Mum loves to try out new things, so she tapped away all week. Her next appointment saw a different outcome. She couldn't wait to tell me that, this time, her tooth came out straight away with no hassle. Mum was so relieved!

*

Through my research, I learned more about how my character may have contributed to my ill-health. In his book, *When the Body Says No. The Cost of Hidden Stress* (2011), Gabor Maté states that:

> Characteristic of many persons with rheumatoid diseases is a stoicism carried to the extreme degree, a deeply ingrained reticence about seeking help. People often put up silently with agonizing discomfort or will not voice their complaints loudly enough to be heard or will resist the idea of taking symptom-relieving medications.[38]

For me, it was that Pollyanna attitude coming into play.

Maté talks of a woman called Celia who was in her thirties (same as me) whose pain was severe. Her girlfriend who had to drive her to emergency asked Celia, 'Do you give up yet?'

'Do you give up yet—what does that mean?' Celia replied.

'I'm stubborn. Whenever I'm sick, I always have this underlying fear that I won't be believed or that I'll be seen as a hypochondriac.'

This way of dealing with illness had been my thought process too, for much of my life.

You think nobody likes a complainer. *Where does this come from?*

Gabor states that 'the non-complaining stoicism exhibited by rheumatic patients is a coping style acquired early in life'.[39]

In *The Subtle Art of not giving a F*ck. A Counterintuitive Approach to Living a Good Life* (2015), Mark Manson states that:

While there is something to be said for "staying on the sunny side of life," the truth is, sometimes life sucks, and the healthiest thing you can do is admit it.[40]

Manson goes on to say that:

Denying negative emotions leads to experiencing deeper and more prolonged negative emotions and emotional dysfunction. Constant positivity is a form of avoidance, not a valid solution to life's problems.[41]

After reading this, my constant "life's good—smiley face—attitude" was challenged.

Manson believes that the trick with negative emotions is to:

1) Express them in a socially acceptable and healthy manner, and

2) Express them in a way that aligns with your values.

This is a great viewpoint. I now write my negative emotions down on paper and this helps me view them and then release them.

How do you translate that to a child?

These days, children are being taught mindfulness and meditation in some schools, and I believe that these are healthy ways of helping them cope in a more peaceful way.

My main lessons would be: *learn to say no when necessary; watch what you eat; be kind to others and yourself; give your brain time to pause; and don't worry, be happy!*

Chapter 9

Reborn

My sun sets to rise again.
—*Robert Browning* [42]

Ihave read that sometimes illness fulfils a positive function in our relationships with others; that children can learn that illness is a sure way to get love and affection from Mum and Dad. [43]

In *Your Mind Power: Strategies for behaviour change* (Stapleton 2007), the chapter entitled, "Engaging your Body's Natural Ability to Heal" by Dr Connirae Andreas, states that love and affection are very important, particularly to young children, and that most people will do whatever they perceive is necessary to get it. Dr Andreas stresses the importance of parents giving their children affection and nurturing when they are well, so that they do not learn that, 'You have to get sick to get love around here.' [44] Others, by contrast, think that it is insulting to believe that they are getting love and attention in this way, so they deny it. It is important to realise that these are positive and useful parts of ourselves. Having ways to experience love, or ways to care for ourselves, are things all of us want. It is only a matter of finding better ways to get these important experiences. While Dr Andreas admits that we should never tell people to give up this method of gaining positive attention, we need to assist each other in 'finding more satisfying ways to get love and affection'.[44]

I was a sickly child and yes, I remember that that was the time when I gained a lot of attention from my two hard working parents. I also wondered if this was connected back to the time of my fall down the stairs at my grandmother's house when I was four or five years of age. I was taken to hospital for stitches in my forehead. My parents were separated at the time, but I had Mum by my bedside.

Reflecting on my unstable life as a child—or at least my childhood where I needed to remain strong through illness, upheaval, injury, and bury my hurts—perhaps seeking more satisfying ways to receive love and care than through illness was what led me on my healing journey.

I have been reborn through Reiki, and I have learned that Reiki energy never leaves you. Even at the oddest moments, I find myself talking to someone when an issue arises in conversation that causes my hands to start heating up and my palms tingle and redden.

You can have fun with Reiki. I remember, one time, going to visit an old friend and his family. His little boy had a toy that he had wanted to play with, but it had stopped running as the batteries had gone flat. I took the batteries out and held them in my hands. I was able to charge them up. We put them back in the toy, and off it went. *Very handy!* You can also have sad times with Reiki. It was our chow chow's eleventh birthday, and my husband had fed him Kentucky chicken as a super treat for his dinner. He bolted it down because he was so excited to be eating this delicious, fatty chicken that he wasn't usually allowed.

Unfortunately, not long after, I could tell our dog was in trouble. I felt him and told my husband to take him to the veterinary hospital. I said, 'He has bloat.' Not wanting to believe me, my husband took him for a walk, trying to get our boy to throw it up. While he was out walking the dog, I rang the hospital. They said to bring our boy in straight away. When my husband came back with from the walk, I told him they were waiting for them. I stayed behind with our other dog and waited for news. The vets confirmed that it was bloat and that he was in pain. The chances were not high that he would make it. My husband came home without our beautiful boy, and this was one time when I wished I had been wrong.

In explaining why I find Reiki and all it entails so easy for me to accept, I must share that I am one of those girls who has always read my weekly horoscope, and I have been going to see clairvoyants since I was a teenager, which is a long time. I am not sure if this is because I need reassuring that my life is on track, or if it is because I have faith in what the universe has to tell me. I feel that I have been blessed by finding my health care angels along my journey to wellness. These angels include the homeopath who diagnosed my polyarthralgia, and, when food was tasting like metal, it was a naturopath who diagnosed that I had mercury leaking from my teeth fillings, so I had all of my amalgam removed. Another naturopath who, after I had gone through twelve years of conventional testing for wheat sensitivity – including swallowing a camera – found that I was wheat intolerant through a simple test, and this really changed my life in a major way. My bodily aches and pains reduced, my skin started glowing, the rashes decreased, and I had so much more energy. Yet another angel was the naturopath who recently found, through MTHFR genetic testing, that I had high food intolerances, which helped put a stop to the anxiety that I had been experiencing for two years.

But, above all, what has worked for me is Reiki, energy work. I have since discovered that many well-known people in the sporting arena and on the stage and screen use these healing modalities. We now know, for example, that Oprah Winfrey and Hugh Jackman practise meditation. It is all about self-care, and what we need to do to heal. These modalities take back our power for our health and wellbeing and can truly help us feel newly born again.

Chapter 10

Share Your Healing

Every moment is a fresh beginning.
—*T S Eliot* [45]

W e all have a story to tell, and there are many stories of miraculous recoveries from trauma and hardships or ill health. This is mine and, although I've had my fair share of illness and injury, I never wanted my health issues to define me.

I want to tell you how all of this came about … me writing this book. I was at the Helensvale library, on the Gold Coast, at a meditation meet and greet, just over three years ago. A rather cute-looking older lady sitting in front turned to me and asked, 'How's your book going?'

I think I gave this sweet lady a blank look and replied, 'What book?'

The lady said, 'Your Reiki book, of course!' Then she gave me her card. She was a clairvoyant.

The funny thing was that, three years prior to this, I had started to write a fictional book about dogs, as we had two gorgeous chow chows, and one of them had provided pet therapy at the local hospices. I had some funny and sad stories from that time that I thought would be good to write about. It was around this time, too, that my husband had a major heart attack.

After that episode, his physician told us that we needed to sell our house. It was a good-sized two storey home, but the stairs were not good for him.

Reluctantly, we put the house on the market, packed away a lot of our personal items, and began holding constant "open home" visits, which meant no time to write that book.

After Kawena, the clairvoyant, told me that I was writing a book on Reiki, I gave it serious thought. *What could I offer readers that could help them?* I decided that, when the time was right, and my body was happy to release its stored trauma through writing, I would write a book on my journey to healing.

Soon after this encounter, I decided I wanted to treat myself. I bought tickets to a Mind Heart Connect Conference to listen to author Joe Dispenza, and another favourite healer of mine Brad Yates, who specialises in EFT tapping. The seminar was being run by Dr Peta Stapleton from Bond University, Queensland. I had used TFT (or EFT as it is now called) back twelve or so years ago when I was first diagnosed as a coeliac disease by a naturopath. It was this practitioner who also showed me how to use the tapping technique.

Another speaker at this conference was Dr David Hamilton, author of *How Your Mind Can Heal Your Body* (2008). Dr Hamilton spoke in his book of the power of positive thinking, explaining that optimists live longer than pessimists (Maruta 2000).[46]

Hamilton referenced a study by the Mayo Clinic in the USA that examined the power of positivity, and its relationship to a longer life. This long-term study ran for 30 years and involved over 400 people and noted their predisposition of being either optimistic or pessimistic. He found that looking on the brighter side of life really did make a difference with optimists having a clear advantage of avoiding an early death over their pessimistic counterparts.[47]

Hamilton wrote that: '… the mind and body are linked while attitude has an impact on the final outcome—death.'[47] Reading Dr Hamilton's words convinced me that my glass half full attitude had served me well throughout my life.

Dr Hamilton explains that:

As we go through our lives, our attitudes affect how we react to viruses, bacteria and other pathogens. A positive, optimistic outlook on life is ultimately better for our overall health and longevity. We also deal with life situations differently depending on our attitude to them. A positive attitude helps us to cope with challenges and even to see them as opportunities which ultimately benefits our health. [47]

It was at the Mind Heart Connect Conference that I also met author and public speaker, Sally Thibault. I told Sally about the time when I was disabled. Thinking back, I must have been feeling safe to have shared this, as it was such a private subject for me, and very few people know of this time in my life. Sally also advised me to write about it. I thought, *If a third person suggests this, then I am going to do it.* I booked in to have a psychic reading, and the book came up yet again. *Alright! Here goes,* I thought, and started to write down my thoughts of that time.

I didn't realise that many issues would come through while trying to put my memories down on paper. I was feeling incredibly vulnerable, and so many questions were coming up while I was writing that, at times, I felt my body almost recreating some of the problems I had endured back then. I felt my brain was screaming, *No! I don't want to go there! Been there, done that, move on.* For some weird reason, fear raised its ugly head and I became scared that I would relapse, and that all that I went through would resurface. So, that was it. No more memoir writing for me. I thought, *Sorry, but I am responsible for me, and who would be interested in my story of chronic illness anyway?*

Then, not long after I had stopped writing, I started having some peculiar health problems. Once again, I was on another path of gaining information and finding different practitioners to help with what was becoming another debilitating problem that was keeping me housebound. This time, my issues were dietary. I was diagnosed with food histamine intolerance. *What is eating at me?* I wondered. *Write the book,* came the answer. I am now on the road to recovery.

Looking back, after receiving the correct diagnosis of EBV, Epstein-Barr Virus, and Cytomegalovirus, I was told that I was eligible for work care payments, as one of these was a virus that I could only contract from where I was working. However, I remained convinced that, as these were just viruses, getting over them would not take long. I treated it as if I had a bad cold, and I believed that I would be back fully functional again, so I stayed on my invalid pension. I have never been sure whether this was my "sliding doors" moment. *Would I have looked for healing alternatives if I did not have money issues?* There's a little saying by Anatole France that goes:

One must never lose time in vainly regretting the past, nor complaining against the changes which cause us discomfort, for change is the very essence of life ...

*

Recently, I attended a book launch at my local library. A local man had written a book about his near-death experience while swimming at the beach. He said he was lucky because the surf lifesaving club had a defibrillator on hand. The lifesavers were able to shock his heart and bring him back to life. The author was campaigning for defibrillators to be installed in supermarkets.

At one stage, the writer asked me what I would do, if someone near me was suffering a heart attack. I shared with him that one Saturday morning, after mowing the back lawn, my husband had suffered a major heart attack. There had never been much grass down there, but, after a considerable downpour, it was now lush and ready for a good mow. My husband came inside, hot and sweaty but pleased with himself for a job well done. Next minute, he fell on the floor in front of me and started pulling off his shirt because he felt unable to breathe. Unfortunately, it was quite serious, yet we didn't know that at the time. Three of his four heart arteries were blocked. My husband was experiencing significant pain, and there was a chance he was about to possibly lose his life. It was daunting for me to see him like this.

I rang for the ambulance and managed to get him to the couch where I started using Reiki on him. It was just automatic. I felt the energy flow through my hands that I placed on his body. I placed my palms each side of his head and, it began to flow through to where it was needed. The paramedics soon arrived. They started working on his chest, and I continued standing at the end of the couch, a short distance away working with the Reiki energy quietly.

My husband has said that while I was performing Reiki on him, it was the only time that he felt any relief from the pain. He said that he could feel the healing energy coming through my hands, and it calmed him.

Luckily for us, our hospital was a short ten-minute drive from home, and they operated on him straight away. The hospital staff had him in for surgery in next to no time, and for that, we are so thankful. That was over five years ago, and my husband has never felt fitter, with his three new titanium stents.

So, when this author asked what I would do, I told him that I did Reiki. While Reiki proved to be the most life-changing healing therapy for me, there are so many healing modalities available to you.

Chapter 11

Your Lifestyle Changes Your Genes

Everything you can imagine is real.
—Pablo Picasso[48]

Traditionally, we may all have learned that our genetic destiny is fixed from birth. However, in his ground-breaking book, *Inheritance: How our Genes Change our Lives—and our Lives Change our Genes* (2014), Dr Sharon Moalem demonstrates that the human genome is far more fluid than we imagined. For example, while you may have recovered from the psychological trauma caused by childhood bullying, Dr Moalem explains that your genes may remain scarred for life.

Everyone agrees that bullying can leave significant mental scars. Dr Moalem goes further, asking, what if our experiences did a lot more? It seems that being bullied can do more damage than we thought. It can change our DNA. Even though we have forgotten, or tried to put it to the back of our minds, or have undergone therapy on this issue and thought all is well, it seems that our genes maintain the trauma adding another stressor to our health. The effects of bullying were tested on sets of twins who had the same genetic makeup. One was bullied, causing significant genetic changes, and one wasn't. The study concluded that bullying changes how our genes work. It changes our stress levels and how we cope.

All the more reason for children to learn mindfulness and kindness at school. Both my brother and sister were bullied at school, and both have the most unusual of health problems today.

Similarly, in her book, *Childhood Disrupted: How your Biography becomes your Biology and how you can Heal* (2015), Donna Jackson Nakazawa states that:

> Cutting-edge research tells us that what doesn't kill you makes you stronger. Far more often, the opposite is true: the early chronic unpredictable stressors, losses, and adversities we face as children shape our biology in ways that predetermine our adult health.[49]

Jackson Nakazawa goes on to talk about the perils of childhood and how it affects our ability to cope with stress as we age and become adults. Jackson Nakazawa believes that, if our childhoods were significantly interrupted, our genes are affected and that we release viruses into our autoimmune system, due to the fact that we are constantly in fight or flight mode. Our coping system, Jackson Nakazawa says, then produces viruses like Epstein-Barr virus and fibromyalgia.

Psychologist Dr Rick Hanson, author of *Hardwiring Happiness: The New Brain Science of Contentment, Calm, and Confidence* (2013), writes about our brain's tendency to have a "negativity bias" and how we readily latch on to negative experiences but find that we seem to ignore or fail to hold on to the positive experiences in our life. This bias may have been useful for the survival of ancient animals, but can cause feelings of loneliness, sadness and anxious in today's busy, modern world.

His book is based on neuroscience and includes a range of methods along with guided practices to help the reader understand the importance of happiness and adjusting their mindset.

The Medical Medium, Anthony William, believes that all mystery illnesses arrive from the Epstein-Barr virus. William writes about the mistaken theory of autoimmune disease. That is, you visit a GP and they give you a diagnosis that you have rheumatoid arthritis. William says, that is just a tag, not an answer. William believes that this autoimmune mystery disease is at an all-time high. You get your prescription for anti-inflammatories. The next thing that happens is that you are put onto a physical therapy program or, as I was, into a pain clinic, and then that is that. The GP gives you no suggestions as to why you have this disease, or how you can heal from it. William provides steps on how to heal yourself, using diet, herbs, and vitamins, some of which I took during my frustrating time of illness.

Further to lifestyle affecting our genes, both Moalem and Pelletier agree that disruptions to individual people's genome, or differences in their DNA, can determine how effective or ineffective certain drugs are, and even our body's reactions to fructose and other foods.

Dr Moalem also states that:

Each year many thousands of people die and many more become acutely ill—precisely because they were taking the exact dosage of medications prescribed to them by their doctors. It's not that their doctors were negligent. In fact, in most cases, their prescriptions were exactly in line with recommendations provided by drug manufacturers and professional medical societies. The reason for many of these adverse drug reactions lies in our genes.[50]

Dr Moalem goes on to explain that it is how much of this gene and how many you have inherited that can lead to different health outcomes. I found the MTHFR reference here and I was glad to read that testing is now being done in hospitals for new Mums-to-be for their individual responses to folic acid.

In his new book, *Change your Genes, Change your Life* (2018), Dr Kenneth R Pelletier[51] integrates a lifetime of research and experiences to distil the new science of how our genes respond to everything we do, and importantly, just how we can use this science to achieve optimal health.

If you're like me, you believed that our genes are static and unchangeable. Dr Pelletier challenges that assumption for, as we now know, what we ingest, breathe, and see, this influences our DNA. A famous example of where genetics impacted a health decision is for actress, Angelina Jolie who, following the death of her mother from breast cancer, had a double mastectomy as a precaution.

In his book, Pelletier states that before 1940 the incidence of breast cancer in women was 24 percent.[51] *What has changed to elevate women's chances more than threefold today? Certainly not the gene itself.* Pelletier explains that the important variables influencing the gene's expression include diet, exercise, exposure to pollutants, and other lifestyle behaviours.

In *Atomic Habits* by James Clear (2018), he demonstrates how transforming your habits maps your biology, and becomes your healing pathway. Sharon Moalem in his books *Inheritance* (2015), goes further, stating that exposure to radiation during flights, ultraviolet radiation from the sun, ethanol in your cocktail, chemical residue in tobacco smoke, insecticides, and chemicals in your personal care products are all examples of general factors that can damage your DNA. He says, 'How you choose to live will determine how well you treat your genome.'[52]

Dr Joe Dispenza, who was told he would never walk again due to his bike accident, states in his book, *Becoming Supernatural. How Common People are doing the Uncommon* (2017), that common people can do the uncommon, and make enormous changes in our health and reverse diseases in our bodies.[53] Dispenza opened up a whole new way of thinking about mind-body health and wellness for me.

Another hero of mine is Australian mining engineer, humanitarian, and athlete, Turia Pitt. Few people could experience burns to sixty-five percent of their body and come out stronger, but Turia is proof it can be done. Turia said in McBride article (2018):

I wish people understood how powerful their mindset was. If you have the right mindset, you can do and be anything you want.[54]

In 2011, the then twenty-four-year-old was competing in an ultra-marathon through Western Australia's Kimberley region when she was caught in a grass fire and suffered horrific burns. Doctors did not expect her to survive. Since then, Turia has undergone hundreds of operations while still competing in events—like the 2016 Ironman World Championships—and she gave birth to her first child in 2017. Now an inspirational speaker and mentor to thousands, Turia shares her healing philosophy in her two books, *Everything to Live For* (2017) and *Unmasked* (2018).

Another author I love is Carolyn Myss who, in her 2017 TED Talk[55], explained that we are continually learning how to observe, and that we have become intrigued with ourselves in a way that other generations have not. Carolyn says that, 'We are the new frontier.' She asks, 'Why do we become ill? Why don't we heal?' Myss thinks it's because we are looking for a story, a narrative, for reasons that are a complexity. Carolyn says we need to put choice as an authority. The power of choice.

A close friend of mine, Madonna—*no, not the superstar!*—said, 'I don't do flu. I have no time for the flu.' Madonna is adamant about this choice. And, guess what? Madonna does not get the flu. I have come to believe that health and healing are the most powerful choices of our lives.

It took me three years to get my health back, but I did it using a plethora of complementary modalities. My journey took many twists and turns as I searched for healing therapies that worked for me. I still have a well-worn, expanded 1988 edition of Louise Hay's, *Heal Your Body: The Mental Causes for Physical Illness and the Metaphysical Way to Overcome them*, which I refer to some thirty years later. I paid $5.95 for mine, and it has become invaluable to me. In her book, Hay explains the relationship between emotional blockages which she believes can lead to physical blockages in the body. Hay outlined the mental causes for physical illness, and the metaphysical way to overcome them.

Hay states:

Take a little time to listen to the words you say. If you hear yourself saying things three times, write it down. It has become a pattern for you. At the end of the week, look at the list you have made, and you will see how your words fit your experiences. Be willing to change your words and thoughts and watch your life change. The way to control your life is to control your choice of words and thoughts. No one thinks in your mind but you.[56]

In 2009, my husband and I had just sold our home in Brisbane, and we were looking to move closer to the Gold Coast as we used to drive for an hour or more to take our dogs walking there. We were looking forward to long walks along the beach and a less stressful lifestyle with cleaner air for us and our two chow chows.

Before deciding on a house to buy, I saw an advertisement for a Hay House weekend seminar in San Diego, titled: 'I Can Do It'. San Diego had always been a city on my bucket list, and here was one of my favourite, dare I say gurus, running a course.

We were visiting the US at the time of the swine flu outbreak, so we had to take all these pills just to be allowed into the country. Many of my favourite authors and healers—Gregg Braden, Wayne Dyer, Bruce Lipton, Dr Brian Weiss, and Denise Linn—were also speaking at the workshop. Their books had been on my shelves at home for well over twenty years and now here I was seeing them in person. Also here was my chance to meet Louise Hay herself and thank her personally for being such an inspiration to me during my time of healing. I felt this was too good an opportunity to miss. *Fantastic!*

After she spoke at the conference, I was queuing to talk to Louise. However, when the time came to meet my idol, I was so tongue-tied I just stuttered my greetings and I did not get to express my thanks to her fully.

Healing from chronic illness or injury is a continuous learning curve. We are constantly updating and upgrading our computers and phones—and the same goes for our health. If only I could turn back the clock thirty years, knowing what I know now about endometriosis and taking the pill, the MTHFR gene, and the folic acid issues with pregnancy, the perils of drinking too much alcohol, and the importance of eating right for good gut and brain health. Luckily, we are finding out so much more there are so many different tools at our fingertips.

Glastonbury Revisited

A couple of years before our trip to the US, my hubby and I flew to the UK. I wanted him to see the country of my birth, and I was curious to see how things had changed in the twenty-five years since I was last there. We were only going to have a short time in England as we wanted to see Paris and some of Spain also. We hired a car and drove to the Cotswolds where we stayed overnight. Then, onto Bath and finally Glastonbury. Because I had an interesting memory of my time there, the first thing we did when reaching Glastonbury was visit the Abbey. While it was nice walking around the grounds of the Abbey, this time I felt no pull, no feeling of wanting to stay.

We were looking for somewhere else to explore, and I thought the Tor might be worth a look. The Tor is a hill with a tower at the top, called St Michael's Tower, which is said to have a lovely view. We parked our car and started the climb along a small path. Suddenly, a surge of despair came over me and I started sobbing. I couldn't move and I was too scared to do the walk.

Other couples were coming down, walking past us. They were probably wondering what was going on because I was on my knees, crying uncontrollably.

*

We headed back down to the car and into the village, so that I could get some tissues and a drink. My husband had pulled the car over to work out where we could park when a lady came up to his window. She told him to pull in to where she was heading and to park in her spot. Then, she said to him, 'Your wife needs help. Take her into the gardens and have her drink from the well inside the grounds.'

How this wonderful angel sensed what was going on with me, we had no idea, but we did as she suggested. We parked the car and walked into the gardens where I drank this brown, metallic-tasting water—it really didn't look too great—from a small well. I started to come good and feel better. We wandered around the grounds and then decided to keep walking to have a look at the local shops. Later, I learnt a lot more about The Tor, the Chalice Well Gardens, and the Red Springs water that I drank. There are incredible legends about these places, as well as the Abbey.

Just prior to our visit, I had watched a fascinating thriller on TV about *The Green Man*. We found a quirky shop in Glastonbury selling books about it. I was wanting a souvenir, so hubby bought me one of these books. As we were paying, the shop owner came up to us and asked if we would like to know more about it. Next thing, he left his shop and took us on a tour down the streets, pointing out to us all the buildings in Glastonbury featuring the Green Man emblem. We were amazed, to say the least, and we felt quite special. *What was this place?* Everyone was so friendly.

We left Glastonbury and decided to miss seeing Stonehenge, as I was still a bit rung-out. We drove on, looking for somewhere to spend the night. A lot of the smaller Bs and Bs were already full, but then I saw a 'vacancy' sign and a long driveway. We pulled in and, at the end, stood a stunning manor. I told hubby that we could only pay a certain amount, so we would see what they had. He came out with a big grin on his face. 'Jan, come and have a look at this,' he said. It seems the only room they had left was called The Oval Room, and it was huge. Believe me, it was bigger than a flat I once rented in Sydney. Not only was this room gorgeous, it was also a third of the price because of the lateness of the evening. Boy, did we get lucky. It was a wonderful way to finish off such an unusual and enlightening day!

Returning home, I was sharing my story with someone about our time in Glastonbury and they said that women were marched up to the Tor and then hung as witches. I have no idea if this is true, but the feelings that I had on that day were of overwhelming grief.

Horstmann Technique

My husband breaches like a whale in bed from back pain. So, in 2004, to stop me from being bounced out of bed which happened once, we traded our comfy mattress and base for a firmer foam mattress and a wooden slat base. It worked well for a time until one night I decided to take a running jump into bed and twisted my spine landing badly. It was incredibly painful for me to move. I was prescribed an anti-inflamma-tory medication by my GP. At that time, it had been on the market for roughly five years, and was being hailed as the new whizz-bang, anti-inflammatory drug.

I started having unusual heart palpitations. I also found that the pills were not having a great deal of effect reducing my pain, so I came off them completely. This turned out to be a wise move as eventually, it was recalled from use.

A specialist suggested that I have nerves deadened in my spine. This was a quick, day procedure, and I gave it a try, twice, approximately three months apart, but it didn't help relieve my pain. I was unable to sit for any length of time, or ride in the car for more than twenty minutes. I can't remember how I found my next healing modality but, somehow, I found a group of women doing a form of healing called the Horstmann technique and, luckily for me, they were just a twenty-minute drive away. After a few sessions with these incredible women, I became not only pain-free, but I was also able to sit in our car while hubby drove us to Coffs Harbour for a holiday, a trip of four hours each way!

,

Chapter 12

Able Me

If my mind can conceive it, and my heart can believe it,
then I can achieve it.
—*Muhammad Ali* [57]

Writing this book has been cathartic for me. It hasn't been easy, but I am so glad I have done it. I want to send out a big thank you to my little angel who first came up to me that day in the library and told me that I would be writing it. Taking on and understanding your illness gives you a why to live, and next comes the how.

When I started to write this book a couple of years ago, it triggered memories in my body. I was like, *Oh, yeah, I remember that*, and then my body started to remember also. I felt so uncomfortable and fearful that I stopped writing. When I looked back to that time when I was incapacitated, it seemed all so daunting. Writing this now, however, I feel more of a release. I remember all the good times that came with the frustration and the pain. The floatation tanks, the peace of taking things slowly sometimes a bit too slowly, the learning, and the interactions with some wonderful practitioners and healers out there.

I am part of a group on Facebook where we talk about health matters because I am still going through healing. As we live and breathe, our bodies change and, as we age, new issues arise.

After reading so many books on the mind-body connection, I can only conclude that my mind told my body, at that time in my life, that enough is enough—stop or slow down, and enjoy being in one place. I wanted to belong to one state, one country, one group of good friends, have one job, and feel connected. My illness ensured that this happened as my body said, stay, in the only way it knew how. As far as I'm concerned, the outcome could not have been better.

These days, I mainly use Reiki on my dogs, and they love it. Animals do, I have found. They are so open to the energy.

We are all individuals, we don't all think or feel the same, but Reiki is the modality that worked for me and, even though I have added to it with other forms of natural healing, it is the one thing, such as when my husband suffered his heart attack, that I start to use without thinking. The energy just flows through me, for whatever was needed at the time.

Reiki bypasses the symptom and goes straight to the core issue, whatever that might be. They say that having a positive attitude is half the battle. Believing is more than half the first and second battle.

In his book, *Hardwiring Happiness* (2013), Rick Hanson explains that our ancestors made two kinds of mistakes: first, in thinking there was a tiger in the bushes when there wasn't one, and second, in thinking there was no tiger in the bushes when there was one. The cost of this, Hanson states, is needless anxiety in the first instance and death in the second. What Rick Hanson was saying is that negativity leads to stress on the body. And what is the pay-off for holding on to the pain? Immobility.

For me, my condition kept me in one place, allowing me to develop long-term friendships and a network of people who got to know me for more than a couple of months. I realised that these friendships were what I came back to Melbourne to find. Quite possibly, after a year or so spent working at the hospital, I would have decided it was time to travel again. My condition made this impossible.

Consistency began to enter my life. Even though it wasn't what I would have chosen in my conscious mind, apparently, I had decided it in my subconscious mind and my body followed suit. I believed that I was destined to remain an invalid, for that amount of time—until I didn't. Yes, we all have these viruses and cancers in our bodies, and numerous triggers can set them off, while others never have these issues.

My message is that you do not have to believe that this is your diagnosis, and you don't have to become a victim of your illness. It is not all cut and dried, but the placebo effect has shown many times that the mind can be your greatest healer. Positive thinking is incredibly powerful.

While medicine and surgery are much needed for trauma, I believe that, for ongoing chronic illnesses, you need alternate therapy healers, together with food/dietary changes, and positive thought patterns. I believe that how you see things—plays a significant role in your recovery from chronic pain and illness.

The value of traditional healing blended with modern practices cannot be overlooked. We can learn so much from the healers with generations of knowledge. An ABC NEWS article in 2019,[58] reported on Aboriginal healers, doctors and nurses working together: "The 60,000-year-old practice involves the use of touch, breath and bush medicine to focus on healing a person's spirit."

To have modern practitioners see the value in healing a person's spirit and tap into ancient healing techniques that resonate so strongly, demonstrates, I believe, how important the health of our mind is in fighting disease and pain in the body. A negative state of mind and belief in ourselves can also greatly affect us, as discussed in Rogers' article, *Primitive Theories of Disease* (1942).[59]

I believe in the biochemistry of love as described by Dr David Hamilton in his book, *How Your Mind Can Heal Your Body: 10th Anniversary Edition* (2018). Dr Hamilton says that, when a person is in an environment where they feel love, thinking about a time when someone showed them love or affection or when they felt close to someone, it could even be an animal, they produce oxytocin hormone in their brain, heart, and reproductive organs. Oxytocin delivers fantastic benefits to the heart, keeping the arteries healthy. It also plays a role in digestion, helping us to digest our food better. I agree with Dr Hamilton that healing can be accelerated when we are thinking of love, compassion, gratitude, affection, kindness, and generosity of spirit.

Many of my major health issues have ultimately been diagnosed by naturopaths, after doctors had exhausted the traditional medicine possibilities. When this happens repeatedly, you do start wondering what is going on. Before I was diagnosed with coeliac disease, I endured ten years of having blood tests for allergies. Then, from another form of test, a naturopath discovered that I was positive to gluten intolerance. I am happy to say I now have both a great GP plus an Integrative Functional Medicine practitioner.

*

I am sitting in a Reiki class—sitting up the back and getting a feel for the energy, enjoying the stories that are being shared by the clients who have just learnt Reiki. They are a warm and caring group, and their hands were activated the previous day. Each of them is being helped with understanding the tool that they now have. An older gentleman shares that he had previously had a stiff neck and used his hands to heal it. When asked why he had a sore neck, the gentleman shares that he was often told that he was "a pain in the neck". He was a funny guy. However, others offered suggestions, including that having a stiff neck could mean that he was unable or unwilling to see what was going on around him, or that his view was limited. The cause will be something for him to work out the meaning for himself, but this caring group offered something that you won't have the privilege to receive if you learn Reiki via DVD. I watch on as another person is being worked on. A tissue has been placed on his face to allow him space and silence without lighting glare. His hand positions are drawing the practitioner's attention, and he explains the meaning behind them. 'Placing the hands on the hips could mean helping with direction or flexibility,' the Reiki practitioner explains. 'Knees are about humility. Having the humility to ask for help.'

The Berlin Wall

My mum had flown down from Katherine in the Northern Territory to visit for her birthday one October. This was during the time when the country was going through a major upheaval with a pilot strike, which had gone on for months in 1989. I had already learnt both Reiki 1 and 2. Recently, Mum reminded me of something we did together at that time that she felt was an amazing experience.

I had taken Mum with me to a Reiki group healing at the centre in South Yarra. Many people had turned up, and the hall was quite full. We had gathered to help with the bringing down of the Berlin Wall. We all sat down, held hands, and sent our healing energy, visualising the wall coming down. Mum said that the feeling in the room was something she couldn't describe and would never forget. Shortly after, the Berlin Wall came down, on November 9th, 1989.

*

This Reiki class was perfect for me. Another time, a young girl was sharing details of her food allergies and, of course, the metaphysical message that come with that, which is eating away at ourselves or a lack of self-worth. I am not saying that once you have the understanding it is all easy peasy, and that I can now eat gluten, but this was a reminder that I needed to love myself more. In group situations, the input from others and your teachers can help you find out what your pain is about, and what your body is telling you. The group setting helps you make that mind-body connection.

The Reiki community is so loving and understanding, and I believe that being part of a community is so important these days, given the disconnect that is happening around us. Even with the street we live in, people do not know their neighbours. That old saying, a problem shared is a problem halved, is true and, perhaps that is why social media is so popular. We look up symptoms, and we share our diagnosis with others. We are taking charge. There are now so many books written and being written about wellness. We put crystals in our water bottles and think nothing of it.

These days kids are being taught meditation and yoga in schools from an early age. *How brilliant is that!* And they are growing vegetables. The awareness is back on our health, their health. I know of one school here in Queensland where they are doing all of that and teaching children kindness, first to themselves, then to others, animals and the environment. A major takeaway is that we tend to look outside of ourselves to find a cure when we are ill when, really, we have it all inside of us.

I am also an advocate of Charlie Goldsmith, another natural healer. Goldsmith believes in whole-body healing. Eating the right foods and certain supplements that are right for him, combined with meditation to use energy from the source, by just sending it. Charlie has a website called *My Good Habits*,[60] and he gives free healings on social media at different times of the month. Energy is all around us, and we draw it into us in many ways. We can draw in energy from the trees around us and the sun, certain movements, prayer, singing, yoga, walking barefoot on the grass, swimming in the ocean, and the list goes on.

The question is: How much time are we willing to give to healing ourselves and maintaining good health?

I am sitting in my kitchen while my house painter is working on changing the colours of our lounge room to lighter and brighter. During the morning, we start a conversation about health issues. It is interesting listening to his beliefs about looking after himself. He needs to keep fit for both his work and for looking after his family. He told me that, while he paints, he listens to podcasts by health professionals from the US about body science. He believes in holding space, and eating well, and drinking protein powders. I was so happy to hear this.

I believe there a link between childhood emotional suppression and physical illness in later life. It certainly seems to be the case in our family. Thinking back, my mum was a child during the Second World War. Mum saw the bombing of her city. Closer to home, the street across the road from where Mum lived was completely flattened—every house was gone. During the Blitz, Mum's family were being bombed both day and night. *Can you imagine what this sort of stress can do to a young child?*

And there is a connection between parents' stressors and the outcomes for their children, whether they are passed down through emotional disconnection between parents and children or combined with, the stressors from a life of poverty, which impact what children eat.

When it comes to food, Dr Pelletier writes, 'At different points over a person's lifetime, we will be able to create a picture of that person's epigenetic state.'[61] One powerful example Pelletier gives is chronic inflammation which contributes to numerous diseases, such as cardiovascular disease, obesity, osteoporosis, cancer, inflammatory bowel disease, asthma, and allergies. He explains that when we include anti-inflammatory foods, like beets, broccoli, nuts, berries, and garlic in our diet, our risk is significantly lowered. Pelletier writes that epidemiological studies, as well as animal experiments, have shown that the maternal diet during pregnancy can produce epigenetic changes through altered methylation in the mother that are inherited by the offspring. That was something I found interesting, due to my recent MTHFR diagnosis.

Book reviewer, Nana, on talking about Pelletier's book, *Change your Genes, Change your Life*, writes that:

> While early life trauma can also cause epigenetic changes, engaging in meditation, social support, and massage, and countering damaging unconscious beliefs can change the way the epigenome functions. Stress—be it biological or psychological—affects every single one of our cells. Yet, so does happiness.[62]

I loved reading that!

Jan Kuperman

Amma, The Hugging Guru

I had taken my husband along with me to many Mind Body Spirit Seminars, but this time we were going to see Amma, the well-known and much loved Indian spiritual leader, known as The Hugging Saint. She was coming to Tallebudgera on the Gold Coast back in 2010, and we were going with another couple, good friends of ours who are interested in trying new things. It turned out to be a long wait. There were so many people queuing for their turn of receiving a hug. My friends gave up and went home. They had a two-hour drive, and it was quite late by this time, getting close to midnight.

Eventually, it was our turn. Amma held us jointly, one on each side. It was all over too soon. We both felt such warmth and a lightness to our being.

Afterwards, my hubby and I shared with each other what we got from the experience.

He said that Amma kept saying to him, 'Midori,' over and over. I said, 'No. You've got it wrong. That's the cocktail liqueur.' He remained adamant that Amma kept telling him to go have a Midori. I have since found out that what Amma was saying was, 'My Darling', or 'My Darling Son'.

How he heard it as Midori, I guess we will never know, or was it just thirst? By this time, we had been sitting, waiting for hours, so put it down to him being a little delirious from tiredness.

Meditation

I wanted to share something that I love doing but, once again, I am not consistent with, which is a shame, but you know my story by now! It is meditation. I have tried many kinds and enjoy listening to Deepak Chopra. I have read of meditation groups who have lowered violence rates. I am sure that you have heard about the Maharishi effect. If not, it is about a group of transcendental meditators who came together to meditate with the intention to bring down the crime rates across twenty-four cities in the United States. They reduced crime by nearly 25%. They did it again in Washington, at a time when there was an upsurge in crime in 1993, and once again the crime rate fell.

The Power of Intention

Lynne McTaggart, the author of *The Intention Experiment* (2008) and *The Power of Eight* (2018), did this with her Peace Intention Experiment with over 11 000 people involved from sixty-five different countries. Thousands of people who took part in the experiment had profound feelings. One person said that they had "a sense of oneness", or as another said, "a welling up of love", and another described it as, "a sense of being pulled into the light". The majority, Lynne writes, reported being "overwhelmed by a surge of compassionate love".[63] What you give out, comes back in more ways than one.

I am writing about this because I live in Australia and, in the 2019-2020 summer, our country experienced the most devastating fires. The bushfires raged for months, and decimated the land, killing many native animals and livestock. Reports claimed that a staggering one billion animals died— unfathomable. An invitation, posted by New Zealand resident Brigeeta Light, went out on social media for users to join in globally to pray for rain in Australia. The date was January 3, 2020. For us here in Queensland, the time was late that Friday afternoon.

I can tell you that it started raining here the very next day. In fact, the rain became torrential, and now we have had an unseasonal amount of heavy rain for the last two months or more. As Brigeeta says, 'Collectively praying/or intending together at the same time, has a much more powerful effect than when we pray individually.'[64] It worked, and all the fires are now out. So, a big thank you to Brigeeta Light, and all who took part.

A collection of people all focused on doing good is so powerful. I have witnessed firsthand what the power of prayer can do within my own family. My cousin was diagnosed with myeloma cancer, which in time proved to be a wrong diagnosis. It was, in fact, stage four lymphoma. He was treated with a new drug that unfortunately closed down his organs, one by one, and was playing havoc with his immune system. He was in hospital for seven very frightening weeks for his family. His church members in Sydney and his family's church in Melbourne started regular prayer sessions for him. His one wish was to see his daughter married. Luckily, this he was able to do. Community and connection are healthy for us.

*

I found my healing modality. I happened upon the right teacher at the right time. Belief is another important piece of the healing puzzle. You need to believe that you are on the right path to health and wellbeing. We are questioning so much more, and we ask more. We go to seminars, we join groups on social media, we look up Doctor Google to help us find answers, and we have a role in our own health and healing. There are so many wonderful healers, doctors, modalities, and books out there for you to try but, please, never give up hope. Set your mind away from the pain, if possible, so that you can think more clearly.

Since writing this book, I have a greater understanding of who I am and why I was someone who would start things, but many times did not follow through. I no longer beat myself up about that, and writing has shown me that I can finish something that is important to me.

I can also say that I have now been living in the same house for the last ten years although, at times, I have had very itchy feet to try somewhere new. But, once again, I feel that staying here was for a reason, and that was to be given the time to write. I had always planned to use what I had learnt, but instead started renovating the houses we were living in, and that became my creative outlet. Writing this book has opened up a whole new Pandora's box, and I have loved what I have learnt along the way and looking back over the choices I have made in my life.

I am so grateful to you for taking the time to read my story and I hope you have been able to find something in it that can help or at least has given you food for thought.

Further Reading

1. All Health Post, *Polyarthralgia Symptoms, Causes, Diagnosis, Treatment*, viewed 17 June 2020, <https://allhealthpost.com/poly-arthralgia>, 2020.

2. Australian Naturopathic Practitioners Association Inc., *What is Naturopathy*? viewed 10 February 2020, https://anpa.asn.au/what-is-naturopathy/, 2020.

3. S Boynton, *Don't let the Turkeys get you Down*, Methuen, US, 1986.

4. J Clear, *Atomic Habits*, Random House, US, 2018.

5. HE Davey, *Japanese Yoga. The way of Dynamic Meditation*, Michi Publishing, Albany, Canada, 2001.

6. J Dispenza, *You Are the Placebo Making Your Mind Matter*, Hay House, London, 2014.

7. J Dispenza, *Becoming Supernatural. How Common People are doing the Uncommon*, Hay House, United States, 2017.

8. S Falck, *What is polyarthralgia?*, Medical News Today, viewed 17 June 2020, <https://www.medicalnewstoday.com/articles/320136#symptoms>, 24 November, 2017.

9. N Goldberg, *Old Friend from Far Away: The Practice of Writing Memoir*, Simon & Schuster, United Kingdom, 2007.

10. C Goldsmith, *My Good Habits*, viewed 11 June 2020, <https://www.mygoodhabits.com/>, 2019.

11. R Halberstein, L DeSantis, A Sirkin, et al., *Healing With Bach® Flower Essences: Testing a Complementary Therapy*, Complementary Health Practise Review, viewed 8 June 2020, SAGE Publications Online, <http://chp.sagepub.com/>, 2007.

12. D Hamilton, *How Your Mind Can Heal Your Body*. Hay House, US, 2008.

13. D Hamilton, *How Your Mind Can Heal Your Body: 10th Anniversary Edition*, Hay House, US, 2018.

14. R Hanson, *Hardwiring Happiness: The New Brain Science of Contentment, Calm, and Confidence,* Harmony Press, US, 2013.
15. L Hay, *You Can Heal Your Life,* Hay House, US, 1984.
16. L Hay, *Heal Your Body,* Hay House, US, 1988.
17. L Holmes, *Supercharge Your Life: How to put real food at the heart of everything.* Murdoch Books, London, 2019.
18. T Honervogt, *The Power of Reiki. An Ancient Hands-On Healing Technique,* St. Martin's Griffin, New York, 2014.
19. T Honervogt, *The Power of Reiki. 2nd Edn,* St. Martin's Griffin, New York, 2014.
20. The John Harvey Gray Center for Reiki Healing, *Miracles Happen Every Day with Reiki!,* viewed 29 January 2020, <https://www.learnReiki.org/everyday-Reiki-miracles/>, 2020.
21. John Hopkins University, Integrative Medicine & Digestive Center, *Reiki,* viewed 29 January 2020, <https://www.hopkins-medicine.org/integrative_medicine_digestive_center/services/Reiki.html>, 2020.
22. D Jackson Nakazawa, *Childhood Disrupted: How your Biography becomes your Biology and how you can Heal,* Simon & Schuster, New York, 2015.
23. K Keyes Jr, *The Hundredth Monkey,* Vision Books, USA, 1982.
24. Love Wide Open's Facebook Group, viewed 6 June 2020, <https://www.facebook.com/groups/375859462835817/>, 2020.
25. M Manson, *The Subtle Art of not giving a F*ck. A Counterintuitive Approach to Living a Good Life,* Pan Macmillan, Australia, 2015.
26. T Maruta, RC Colligan, M Malinchoc, KP Offord, *Optimists vs. Pessimists: Survival Rate among Medical Patients over a 30-year period,* Mayo Clinic Proceedings, No. 75, p. 140-143, 2000.
27. G Maté, When *the Body Says No. The Cost of Hidden Stress,* Penguin, UK, 2019.
28. G McBride, *Life Lessons from people who've faced death: Turia Pitt,* NIB, viewed 11 June 2020, <https://www.nib.com.au/the-checkup/community/life-lessons-turia-pitt>, 8 August, 2018.
29. L McTaggart, *The Intention Experiment,* Harper Element, London, UK, 2007.
30. *Connecting and healing with the Power of Eight®,* Facebook Group, viewed 11 June 2020, <https://www.facebook.com/groups/1068844430161141/>, 2020.

31. L McTaggart, *Lynne McTaggart,* viewed 11 June 2020, <https://lynnemctaggart.com/>, 2020.

32. L McTaggart, *The Power of Eight*, Atria Press, US, p. 87, 19 November 2018.

33. S Moalem, *Inheritance: How our Genes Change our Lives—and our Lives Change our Genes*, Grand Central Publishing, London, UK, 2014.

34. C Myss, Trans. S Pangambam, *Choices that can change your Life*, TEDx Findhorn Salon, viewed 10 February 2020, https://singjupost.com/caroline-myss-choices-that-can-change-your-life-at-tedxfindhornsalon-transcript/>, 27 April, 2017.

35. K Noonan Gores, *Heal,* Beyond Words Publishing, New York, 2019.

36. N Ortner, *The Tapping Solution for Pain Relief.* Hay House, US, 2015.

37. N Ortner, *The Tapping Solution*, viewed 17 February, 2020, <https://www.thetappingsolution.com/about-nick-ortner/>, 2020.

38. KR Pelletier, *Change your Genes, Change your Life: Creating Optimal Health with the New Science of Epigenetics.* Origin Press, San Rafael, CA, July 2018.

39. C Parker, *One Soul, Many Faces: Revealing The Hidden Truth: Bringing All Religions & Humanity Back To (The Source) Oneness of God!* CreateSpace Independent Publishing Platform, Kindle, 2013.

40. T Pitt, *Everything to Live For,* Penguin, UK, 2017.

41. T Pitt, *Unmasked,* Random House, US, 2018.

42. J Pizzorno 2018, *The Toxin Solution,* HarperCollins, New York, 2018.

43. C Pullen, *Post World War II British Migration to Australia,* viewed 05 June 2020, <https://collections.museumsvictoria.com.au/articles/13640>, 2014.

44. A Ross, *Genes and Environment in BRCA-Positive Breast Cancer,* ARC Journal of Cancer Science, viewed 17 June 2020, <www.arcjournals.org>, vol. 1, p.17-19, 2015.

45. A de Saint-Exupéry, *The Little Prince*, Penguin, UK, 1998.

46. G Sandwall, *Welcome to Reiki.nu — Reiki — You Can Do It!* viewed 10 February 2020, <www.Reiki.nu>, 2009.

47. P Stapleton ed, *Your Mind Power: Strategies for behaviour change*, Hybrid Press, p. 118. 2007.

48. N Servant, A McConnell, *Historical Heritage of the Apple Industry in* The Commonwealth of Australia, *Tasmania; A Profile. December 1999, Report of the Queen Victoria Museum and Art Gallery,* Launceston, December 1999.

49. D Stein, *Essential Reiki.* Crossing Press, New York, 1995.

50. D Stein, *Essential Reiki Workshop.* DVD. Crossing Press, US, 2007.

51. C Tran, *Paleo diet advocate Pete Evans responds to the growing push for plant-based food – and says his health deteriorated to the 'worst it's ever been' after being vegan for four years,* Daily Mail Australia, published 21 November 2019, viewed 10 June 2020, <https://www.dailymail.co.uk/femail/article-7708193/Paleo-Pete-Evans-reveals-REALLY-thinks-plant-based-vegan-diet.html>, 2019.

52. F Tuck, *Histamine Intolerance*, King Street Press, viewed 10 June 2020,<https://www.fionatuck.com/post/2017/06/05/histamine-intolerance>, 2017.

53. US Department of Health & Human Services, Centers for Disease Control and Prevention, *Adverse Childhood Experiences Study,* viewed 9 June 2020, <https://www.cdc.gov/violenceprevention/childabuseandneglect/acestudy/ace-brfss.html>, 2020.

54. A William, *Medical Medium: Secrets Behind Chronic and Mystery Illness and how to finally Heal,* Hay House Inc, 2015.

55. A William, *Liver Rescue.* Hay House Inc, US, 2018.

56. B Yates, *Tap with Brad. Feel Better, Do Better, Live Better,* viewed 9 June 2020, <https://tapwithbrad.mykajabi.com/>, 2020.

57. Y Ykelenstam, *Healing Histamine,* viewed 10 June 2020, <https://healinghistamine.com/>, 2017.

58. A Zaffarano Rowland, *The Complete Book of Traditional Reiki. Practical Methods for Personal and Planetary Healing.* Inner Traditions Bear and Company, Rochester, VT, USA, 2010.

Additional Information

I have listed the people and organisations that I have found to be helpful along my healing path.

Brad Yates: Tapping with Brad: A free weekly tapping session; https://www.tapwithbrad.com/why-eft/

Charlie Goldsmith: My Good Habits: https://www.mygoodhabits.com/

Deepak Chopra with Oprah Winfrey: Online Meditations: https://chopracentermeditation.com/

Don Tolman: Wholefoods: https://tolmanselfcare.com/

Donna Eden: Kinesiology: https://edenenergymedicine.com

Dr David Perlmutter; https://www.drperlmutter.com

Goop: A Great Wellness Section: https://goop.com/

Dr Ben Lynch: https://www.drbenlynch.com/

Dr Joe Dispenza: https://drjoedispenza.com/

Dr Josh Axe: https://draxe.com/

Dr Peta Stapleton: https://petastapleton.com/

Hermann Müller: http://www.psychosomatictherapycollege.com.au/

Jack Lim: www.relaxationmusic.com.au

Ian White: Australian Bush Flower essences: https://ausflowers.com.au/

Lissa Rankin: www.lissarankin.com

Lynne McTaggart: Online group healings: https://lynnemctaggart.com/experience-your-own-healing-power-of-eight-group/

Medical Medium: Anthony William on Facebook for free health information: https://www.facebook.com/medicalmedium/

MTHFR Support Australia:

https://mthfrsupport.com.au/2016/09/histamine-and-gut-health-the-unlikely-connection-between-allergies-and-our-own-gut-microbes/

Mind Valley Academy: https://www.mindvalley.com/

Sally Thibault: https://www.sallythibault.com.au/

Scott Alexander King: https://animaldreaming.com/

The Heal group: http://www.heal.com.au/

Yasmina Ykelenstam: Best source for recipes and information on what supplements will help with high histamine food intolerance: https://healinghistamine.com/

List of References

1. *Love Wide Open's* Facebook Page, accessed 6 June 2020, <https://www.facebook.com/groups/375859462835817/>
2. N Goldberg, *Old Friend from Far Away: The Practice of Writing Memoir*, Simon & Schuster, United Kingdom, p. 297, 2007.
3. *Connecting and healing with the Power of Eight®*, Facebook Group, viewed 11 June 2020, <https://www.facebook.com/groups/1068844430161141/>
4. Oxford Reference (2020), *Oxford Essential Quotations*, viewed on 27 July 2020, <https://www.oxfordreference.com/view/10.1093/acref/9780191826719.001.0001/q-oro-ed4-00005287>
5. Penn State University (2020), *Quote Analysis*, viewed on 27 July 2020, <https://sites.psu.edu/marissanicolespassionblog/2013/11/01/go-confidently-in-the-direction-of-your-dreams-live-the-life-you-have-imagined-%E2%80%A8-henry-david-thoreau/>
6. C Pullen, *Post World War II British Migration to Australia*, Museums Victoria Collections, 2014, viewed 05 June 2020, <https://collections.museumsvictoria.com.au/articles/13640>
7. Your Dictionary (2020), *Theodore Roosevelt Quotes*, viewed on 27 July 2020, <https://quotes.yourdictionary.com/author/theodore-roosevelt/611085>
8. N Servant, A McConnell, *Historical Heritage of the Apple Industry in* The Commonwealth of Australia, *Tasmania; A Profile. December 1999, Report of the Queen Victoria Museum and Art Gallery*, Launceston, December 1999.
9. R Halberstein, L DeSantis, A Sirkin, et al., *Healing With Bach® Flower Essences: Testing a Complementary Therapy*, Complementary Health Practise Review, viewed 8 June 2020, SAGE Publications Online, <http://chp.sagepub.com/>
10. Poetry Foundation (2020), *In a Dark Time*, viewed on 27 July 2020, <https://www.poetryfoundation.org/poems/43347/in-a-dark-time>
11. K Noonan Gores, *Heal*, Beyond Words Publishing, New York, p. 171, 2019.
12. S Boynton, *Don't let the Turkeys get you Down*, Methuen, US, 1986.
13. University of California, Los Angeles (2020), *They Say Einstein Said*, viewed on 27 July 2020, <http://web.cs.ucla.edu/~klinger/tenpp/11_einstein.html>
14. C Parker, *One Soul, Many Faces: Revealing The Hidden Truth: Bringing All Religions & Humanity Back To (The Source) Oneness of God!* Kindle edn, CreateSpace Independent Publishing Platform, 2013.

15 Movie Quote DB (2020), *The Wizard of Oz Quotes*, viewed on 27 July 2020, <https://www.moviequotedb.com/movies/wizard-of-oz-the/views.html>

16 The John Harvey Gray Center for Reiki Healing, *Miracles Happen Every Day with Reiki!*, viewed 29 January 2020, <https://www.learnReiki.org/everyday-Reiki-miracles/>

17 John Hopkins University, Integrative Medicine & Digestive Center, *Reiki*, viewed 29 January 2020, <https://www.hopkinsmedicine.org/integrative_medicine_digestive_center/services/Reiki.html>

18 Zaffarano Rowland, *Amy, The Complete Book of Traditional Reiki. Practical Methods for Personal and Planetary Healing*, Inner Traditions Bear and Company, Rochester, VT, USA, p. 42, 2010.

19 K Keyes Jr, *The Hundredth Monkey*, Vision Books, USA, 1982.

20 H E Davey, *Japanese Yoga. The way of Dynamic Meditation*, Michi Publishing, Albany, Canada, p. 29, 2001.

21 Australian Naturopathic Practitioners Association Inc., *What is Naturopathy?* viewed 10 February 2020, <https://anpa.asn.au/what-is-naturopathy/>

22 R Halberstein, L DeSantis, A Sirkin, et al., *Healing With Bach® Flower Essences: Testing a Complementary Therapy*, Complementary Health Practise Review, viewed 8 June 2020, SAGE Publications Online, <http://chp.sagepub.com/>

23 G Maté, *When the Body Says No. The Cost of Hidden Stress*, Penguin, UK, p. 57, 2019.

24 N Ortner, *The Tapping Solution for Pain Relief, A Step-by-step Guide to Reducing and Eliminating Chronic Pain*, Hay House, US, p. 118, 2013.

25 US Department of Health & Human Services, Centers for Disease Control and Prevention, *Adverse Childhood Experiences Study*, viewed 9 June 2020, <https://www.cdc.gov/violenceprevention/childabuseandneglect/acestudy/ace-brfss.html>

26 B Yates, *Tap with Brad. Feel Better, Do Better, Live Better*, viewed 9 June 2020, <https://tapwithbrad.mykajabi.com/>

27 G Sandwall, *Welcome to Reiki.nu — Reiki — You Can Do It!* viewed 10 February 2020, <www.Reiki.nu>

28 A de Saint-Exupéry, *The Little Prince*, Penguin, UK, p. 72, 1988.

29 A William, *Medical Medium: Secrets Behind Chronic and Mystery Illness and how to finally Heal*, Hay House Inc, p. 253, 2015.

30 A William, *Medical Medium: Secrets Behind Chronic and Mystery Illness and how to finally Heal*, Hay House Inc, p. 254, 2015.

31 J Pizzorno, *The Toxin Solution*, HarperCollins, New York, p. 109, 2018.

32 J Pizzorno, *The Toxin Solution*, HarperCollins, New York, p. 209, 2018.

33 F Tuck, *Histamine Balance: Is your Superfood Overdose the Culprit behind your itching eyes, skin rashes and troubled sinuses?* The Courier-Mail, Murdoch Press p. 61, 2020.

34 F Tuck, *Histamine Intolerance*, King Street Press, viewed 10 June 2020, <https://www.fionatuck.com/post/2017/06/05/histamine-intolerance>

35 Y Ykelenstam, *Healing Histamine*, viewed 10 June 2020, <https://healinghistamine.com/>

36 C Tran, *Paleo diet advocate Pete Evans responds to the growing push for plant-based food — and says his health deteriorated to the 'worst it's ever been' after being vegan for*

four years, Daily Mail Australia, published 21 November 2019, viewed 10 June 2020, <https://www.dailymail.co.uk/femail/article-7708193/Paleo-Pete-Evans-reveals-REALLY-thinks-plant-based-vegan-diet.html>

37 L Holmes, *Supercharge Your Life: How to put real food at the heart of everything*, Murdoch Books, US, 2019.

38 G Maté, *When the Body Says No. The Cost of Hidden Stress*, Penguin, UK, p. 170, 2019.

39 G Maté, *When the Body Says No. The Cost of Hidden Stress*, Penguin, UK, p. 171, 2019.

40 M Manson, *The Subtle Art of not giving a F*ck. A Counterintuitive Approach to Living a Good Life,* Pan Macmillan, Australia, p. 17, 2015.

41 M Manson, *The Subtle Art of not giving a F*ck. A Counterintuitive Approach to Living a Good Life,* Pan Macmillan, Australia, p. 84, 2015.

42 Quotes of Famous People (2020), *My Sun Sets to Rise Again*, viewed on 27 July 2020, <https://quotepark.com/quotes/960400-robert-browning-my-sun-sets-to-rise-again/>

43 P Stapleton ed, *Your Mind Power: Strategies for behaviour change*, Hybrid Press, p. 118, 2007.

44 P Stapleton ed, *Your Mind Power: Strategies for behaviour change*, Hybrid Press, p. 118, 2007.

45 T S Eliot (2020), *Popular Quotes Attributed to T.S. Eliot*, viewed on 27 July 2020, <http://tseliot.sites.luc.edu/quotes.php>

46 T Maruta, RC Colligan, M Malinchoc, KP Offord, *Optimists vs. Pessimists: Survival Rate among Medical Patients over a 30-year period*, Mayo Clinic Proceedings, No. 75, p. 140-143, 2000.

47 D Hamilton, *How Your Mind Can Heal Your Body*, Hay House, US, p. 5, 2018.

48 Quodid (2020), *The Ultimate Quotation Repository*, viewed on 27 July 2020, <http://quodid.com/quotes/7900/pablo-picasso/everything-you-can-imagine-is-real>

49 D Jackson Nakazawa, *Childhood Disrupted: How your Biography becomes your Biology and how you can Heal*, Simon & Schuster, New York, p. xiii, 2015.

50 S Moalem, *Inheritance: How our Genes Change our Lives—and our Lives Change our Genes*, Grand Central Publishing, London, UK, Kindle edn, 2014.

51 KR Pelletier, *Change your Genes, Change your Life: Creating Optimal Health with the New Science of Epigenetics,* Origin Press, San Rafael, CA, July 2018.

52 S Moalem, *Inheritance: How our Genes Change our Lives—and our Lives Change our Genes*, Grand Central Publishing, London, UK, p. 174, 2014.

53 J Dispenza, *Becoming Supernatural. How Common People are doing the Uncommon.* Hay House, United States, p. iii, 2017.

54 G McBride, *Life Lessons from people who've faced death: Turia Pitt*, NIB, viewed 11 June 2020, <https://www.nib.com.au/the-checkup/community/life-lessons-turia-pitt>

55 C Myss, Trans. S Pangambam, *Choices that can change your Life*, TEDx Findhorn Salon, viewed 10 February 2020, <https://singjupost.com/caroline-myss-choices-that-can-change-your-life-at-tedxfindhornsalon-transcript/>

56 L Hay, *Heal Your Body. The Mental Causes for Physical Illness and the Metaphysical Way to Overcome them*, Hay House, US, p. 4, 1988.

[57]   Your Dictionary (2020), *Muhammed Ali Quotes*, viewed on 27 July 2020, <https://quotes.yourdictionary.com/author/muhammad-ali/21385>

[58]   Rhett Burnie, *Aboriginal healers treat patients alongside doctors and nurses at Lyell McEwin Hospital*, viewed 7 July 2020, <https://www.abc.net.au/news/2019-02-20/aboriginal-healers-treat-patients-alongside-doctors-and-nurses/10826666>

[59]   Spencer L. Rogers, *Primitive Theories of Disease*, Ciba Symposium, Vol. 4, No. 1, April, 1942.

[60]   C Goldsmith, *My Good Habits*, viewed 11 June 2020, <https://www.mygoodhabits.com/>

[61]   KR Pelletier, *Change your Genes, Change your Life: Creating Optimal Health with the New Science of Epigenetics,* Origin Press, San Rafael, CA, p.54, July, 2018.

[62]   C Nana, *Book Review: Change your Genes, Change your Life,* Psychology Central Reviews, viewed 17 June 2020, <https://psychcentralreviews.com/2019/book-review-change-your-genes-change-your-life/>

[63]   L McTaggart, *The Power of Eight®,* Atria Press, US, p. 87, 19 November 2018.

[64]   B Light, *Worldwide Collective Prayer Invitation for Australia*, viewed 11 June 2020, <https://www.facebook.com/brighdelight>